GW00716992

HOUSING FOR HEALTH

Edited by

Susan J. Smith

Department of Geography
University of Edinburgh

Ann McGuckin

Department of Geography
University of Edinburgh

Robin Knill-Jones

Department of Public Health
University of Glasgow

LONGMAN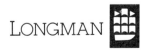

HOUSING FOR HEALTH

Longman Group UK Limited, Longman Industry and
Public Service Management Publishing Division
Westgate House, The High, Harlow, Essex CM20 1YR

First published 1991

A catalogue record for this book is available from the British Library

ISBN 0-582-07832-6

Printed and bound in Great Britain by
Biddles Limited, Guildford and King's Lynn

Contents

Contents

Part II Housing provision for 'medical needs'

Contents

Method
Outcome measures
Professional autonomy
Findings from the study
Services provided and use of the schemes
Problems and difficulties
Achievements
Recommendations

Preface and acknowledgements

The works collected in this book have a common aim: to illustrate the importance of housing provision in the promotion of good health, the prevention of disease, and the delivery of care and support to those who are ill. This role for housing as an instrument of health care, or as an element of social policy more broadly, is not popular in today's political and economic climate. Instead, for at least fifteen years, the thrust of housing policy has been to replace the state by the market, and to emphasise the role of home ownership in fostering Britain's development as a property owning democracy.

Amid the excitement of these developments, it is easy to lose sight of the question 'What do we want housing policy to achieve in a socially just society?' Yet, an informed answer to that question will urge that housing should be more than simply a piece of private property that represents a reasonable investment, an appreciating asset, and a source of cheap housing services in old age. These features are not unimportant, but a key achievement of British social policy in the post-war years was to make housing a cornerstone of the welfare state. Housing provision was seen as a means of offsetting in kind some of the disadvantages and inequalities that necessarily accrue from a market economy. The housing service, like the health service, was regarded as a basic citizenship entitlement, and the role of housing and rehousing in securing decent homes for people with health problems was undisputed.

Currently, both housing and health care policy are undergoing a radical change. This is part of a more general pattern of welfare restructuring in Britain, and in other parts of the developed world. Any form of reorganisation and readjustment includes losers as well as winners. However, most would agree that in a civilized society, people with health problems or medical needs — ordinary people whose incomes may be depressed and whose needs may be increased for reasons largely beyond their control — should be the last to lose out. This book considers whether, in the turmoil of the late twentieth century, it is as easy as we might think for people with medical needs to find appropriate, affordable homes and to secure adequate health care and social support without compromising their residential choice.

The idea for this book grew from a conference on housing and health convened jointly by the Centre for Housing Research, the Department of Public Health, and the MRC Medical Sociology Unit at Glasgow University. The editors are grateful to participants for providing a lively debate and a seedbed of rich ideas — ideas which we have attempted to nurture in designing the present volume. We would also like to acknowledge Dr Sheila MacIver's contribution to this work. Sheila was involved in organising the conference and in developing the outline for the book, but moved on to other things, and was unable to take on the role of an editor. We are also grateful to Dr Mike Summerfield for help in finalising the manuscript.

Susan J. Smith
Ann McGuckin
Robin Knill-Jones

Contributors

Isobel Allen	Capita PLC
David Clapham	Centre for Housing Research, University of Glasgow
Jim Connelly	Department of Public Health Medicine, University of Leeds
Jean Conway	School of Urban and Regional Studies, Sheffield City Polytechnic
Sarah Curtis	Department of Geography, Queen Mary and Westfield College, University of London
Karen Hancock	Centre for Housing Research, University of Glasgow
Robin Knill-Jones	Department of Public Health, University of Glasgow
Ann McGuckin	Department of Geography, University of Edinburgh
Peter Molyneux	AIDS and Housing Project
Jenny Morris	Freelance Researcher
Roz Pendlebury	AIDS and Housing Project
Simon Ramsden	Great Chapel Street Medical Centre and Wytham Hall Sick Bay
Paul Roderick	Department of Public Health Medicine, North-West Thames Regional Health Authority
Nigel Shanks	Accident and Emergency Services,King Khalid Hospital, Jeddah

Susan J. Smith   Department of Geography,
                       University of Edinburgh

Paul Spicker   Department of Political Science and
                       Social Policy, University of Dundee

Rick Stern   Single Homeless Health Action
                       Research Project

Barbara Stilwell   Single Homeless Health Action
                       Research Project

Sandra Williams   Policy Studies Institute

1 Introduction

Ann McGuckin and
Susan J. Smith

Is housing policy good for your health?

The relevance of housing to an understanding of health and welfare has never seriously been in doubt. Nevertheless, the response of policy makers and politicians to this link has varied over the years. In the late nineteenth century, under the auspices of the Ministry of Health, housing issues were at the core of the public health movements and health concerns were a centre-piece of the earliest housing policies. The 'problem' at this time was the extent of unhealthy housing in the major cities, and the 'solutions' were sought not only in public health legislation but also in housing interventions like the *Artisans' and Labourers' Dwellings Act (1868)* and the *Housing of the Working Classes Act (1898)*. These early housing policies are documented by Malpass and Murie (1987). The question that preoccupied policy makers was 'does housing affect health?'. Where the answer was 'yes', a range of mechanisms were put in place to close, demolish or improve unfit properties.

The advent of slum clearance (in the 1930s and again in the 1950s) brought with it an assumption that the demolition of old and unfit stock would largely eradicate the housing related health inequalities of the earlier part of the century. For some sick people, the process of vacating unhealthy homes was further hastened by the development, within the newly constructed public rented sector, of housing management practices which allowed priority in the process of rehousing slum dwellers to be given to people with medical needs. Thus sick people moved more quickly than average from the inner cities to the peripheral estates and new town developments, and the role of housing provision as an instrument of health care was born.

In the interim, it has become apparent that much modern housing is itself a health hazard for some occupants. Slum clearance was never the panacea that politicians hoped for. The extent of damp, cold, mould, overcrowding, and poor repair has once again raised

1

some 'traditional' questions relating to the health effects of dwelling condition (as well as focusing attention on the potential health gains of housing improvements). Some of this work is reviewed in Smith (1989). As much as 15 per cent of the housing stock is in poor repair (Department of the Environment 1988) rising to 85 per cent in the council rented sector (Audit Commission 1986). Up to 1.5 million homes are now unfit for occupation or lack basic amenities (Niner 1990) and around 2.5 million homes suffer dampness. Two million of these home are 'severely' damp (Building Research Establishment 1986)—a condition most often implicated in a range of respiratory problems in adults and, especially, children (Curtis and Hyndman 1989; Hyndman 1990; Martin et al 1987; Platt et al 1989; Strachan and Elton 1986; Strachan and Sanders 1989). There is, then, scope for much more research and thinking on this theme, which is now being taken up by the Healthy Cities Initiative and by local pressure groups like the Right to Warmth Campaign (Sheldrick 1988).

The papers collected in this volume acknowledge the critical effect of housing conditions on occupants' health, but they place most emphasis on two themes which have, so far, been strangely neglected in the resurgence of interest in the links between housing provision and health needs.

The first theme is concerned with the more 'traditional' question: **Does housing affect your health?**. However, authors tackling this issue are concerned not only with the adverse effects of poor living conditions but also with the health problems that might be linked to inadequate access to health care services. This first question does, therefore, probe the links between adverse housing environments and the incidence of certain physical diseases and mental illnesses. However, the authors also take a wider view, documenting the extent to which access to different parts of the housing stock (which varies in quality, desirability and accessibility) are implicated in the reproduction of health inequalities, simply because housing acts as a gateway to health service delivery. This topic is addressed by the essays in part one, and it is also a theme at the heart of part three, which shows just how important it is simply to have a home in order to gain access to the caring services.

The second question tackled in this volume turns attention away from the direct role of housing in conferring health inequalities and towards the potential role of housing policy as an instrument of health care. Housing may reproduce health inequalities, but housing provision could also act as a point of intervention in the cycle of health inequality. This second theme therefore centres around the question **'Does your health affect your housing opportunities?'**. In part two of this volume the authors address this question. Their starting point is the general assumption that, in a society like Britain, if housing provision interacts with health status at all, it will do so to the relative advantage of sick people. Broadly, the social contract might, in theory, dictate that people in poor health should find homes in the more 'healthy' segments of the housing stock. In fact, the findings of part two (and many of the chapters in part three) challenge some conventional assumptions about the welfare ideal, raising the uncomfortable possibility that rather than affording sick people access to healthy environments, the markets and institutions of the housing system might in effect 'select' such people into some of the *worst* parts of the housing stock. Some reappraisal of the social role of housing policy is clearly required if this position is to change.

Although they may appear to address quite distinct issues and policy areas, these questions—focusing on the link between housing and health, and on the consequences of health for housing opportunities—are two sides of a single coin. When, where and how we tackle each of them ultimately depends on what role society sees for housing policy at a particular time. If housing policy is regarded as an instrument of urban revitalisation, then interventions will most obviously be directed towards 'curing' unhealthy homes. From this perspective, the costs of housing improvements can be set (amongst other things) against their public health benefits and against any associated savings to health service budgets. Where housing provision is more closely aligned to the interests of social policy, the emphasis will be placed on the role of housing management as a health care service: on the potential health benefits of rehousing, on the packaging of housing schemes with health care and social support, and on the link between housing management and health care servicing.

In practice, the various strands of housing policy tend to coexist, although one element may be more dominant than another during particular periods and in different political climates (Clapham et al 1990). Moreover, the two roles already mentioned—housing as an element of both urban and social policy—have to be negotiated alongside the use of housing policy as an instrument of economic management. This latter use has dominated in recent years and it may, in the present decade at least, compromise the value of the other two, at least with respect to the housing opportunities available to people with health needs (a point discussed in chapter four).

Housing as a gateway to public health

The papers collected in this volume span both the main approaches to the links between housing and health that are

3

outlined above. Part 1 addresses the first approach and contains two chapters which are concerned with the spatial inequalities in access to health care which flow from the procedures used to allocate health care resources. It is because the availability and quality of health services varies in space that dwelling location affects access to health care. It is because housing is itself an uneven resource that social inequalities are mapped onto the residential environment. And it is because the health services are generally less available to people in the poorest urban areas that inequalities in housing and in access to health care become aligned (though, as MacIntyre (1989) shows, it is much more difficult to confirm the next step in this argument, ie that health care inequalities are implicated in health inequalities overall).

Sarah Curtis is concerned in the second chapter to document the range of factors mediating between residential location and health service availability. The problems of specifying these links are compounded by the difficulty of measuring characteristics like 'need', 'quality of care', and the health 'outputs' of particular services. The task is compounded further by the fundamental problem of defining just what a health care service is or should be. Nevertheless Curtis' outline of the principles used for allocating health care resources reveals some crucial problems in the formulae developed by the Resource Allocation Working Party (RAWP) (which was formed during 1976 to address the question of regional inequalities in the distribution of health expenditure). Shortcomings in the formulae (which use standardised mortality ratios (SMRs) as a proxy for health care need) may prevent the district health authorities from adequately performing their new roles and responsibilities (especially in the area of community care). This is acknowledged in the 1989 white paper *Working for Patients* (Cm 555, (1989), which recommends a new approach, but as Carr-Hill et al (1990) show, it is by no means clear that an appropriate measure of need will be built into this.

Perhaps Curtis' most penetrating analysis comes in a consideration of the factors affecting health care provision from area to area at a local level. Here, she points to the fundamental importance of housing provision as an element of local health care strategies (especially where such provision forms a link between deinstitutionalization and access to community care). Equally crucially, she argues that both the fact of securing permanent accommodation (as distinct from being homeless) and the location of that accommodation are important for gaining access to many parts of the primary health care services. Although there is mixed evidence that an 'inverse care law' is at work, it is still the case that the inner cities which largely contain the older and worst quality housing, and comprise the poorer segments of the city, are dominated

4

by older doctors working alone (rather than in a health centre or large practice) and by relatively old, poorly maintained hospitals without 'state of the art' equipment.

In Chapter 2, Karen Hancock builds on this overview and examines in more detail the problem of resource allocation in the National Health Service through the RAWP formulae. She argues that the key difficulty with these formulae is that social factors, including housing conditions, may be a better proxy for morbidity (and therefore for health care demand) than the SMRs currently used. She shows, for instance, that although the national resource allocation formula is unable to respond to the incidence of unhealthy housing, patients' housing conditions may be an important factor influencing demand for and use of hospital resources. She stresses that local needs indicators are currently inconsistent with those in the national formula. However, she also points out that, although there has of late been little formal link between housing and health policy, changes associated with the current NHS review may cause resource allocation to become more sensitive not only to clinical criteria but also to variations in local housing and social conditions. In practice, if the most appropriate measures are chosen for the resource allocation procedures, the formal contribution of adverse housing conditions to securing funds for health service provision might actually increase.

Health as a gateway to housing opportunities

Part II goes on to show that while housing outcomes may place important constraints on access to health care provision, also health can be an important determinant of housing opportunities. An overview of the main issues is provided in Chapter 4 which also argues for a more systematic programme of research and policy evaluation aiming to specify and respond to the housing needs of people with a wide range of health problems.

Some elements of that programme are developed in chapters five to nine. These chapters are all broadly concerned with the strengths and limitations of using housing provision as an instrument of health care. Although this element of housing policy is rarely analysed in detail, it has played an influential role in British social policy during the last half century. Indeed, public housing was a cornerstone of the welfare state and for many years housing management practices have offered sick people considerable priority in the queue for subsidized accommodation. This practice is founded on the broadly egalitarian view that the state should offer some compensation—in cash or kind—to those unable to compete for market resources in a capitalist economy.

Over the last decade, the stock of council housing—the main vehicle in the housing system by which progressive welfare transfers are made—has been reduced in absolute terms by a policy of sales to sitting tenants, and by a virtual halt on newbuild. Sales have also been selective: the better dwellings have been sold to the higher income tenants of longer standing. Overall, the stock of council housing has diminished in quality as well as size, and the population of council tenants has shifted further down the income scale and is increasingly dominated by families who are dependent on benefits. This process of 'residualization' is now well documented in the housing literature, but is perhaps best summarized in Forrest and Murie (1988).

The increasing economic marginality of council tenants is as much a reflection of the lack of affordable housing outside the public sector as it is a positive choice to rent. This means that people with medical needs are increasingly queueing alongside people with other urgent needs and claims to housing priority (made on the basis of homelessness, local connections, overcrowding and so on). Some of the consequences of this for the organization and viability of using medical priority as a criterion in housing allocations decisions are discussed by Jim Connelly and Paul Roderick in Chapter 5.

Connelly and Roderick assess the rationale underpinning the so-called medical priority system, which, despite the long association between housing provision and public health policy, is today the primary focus of medical involvement in housing issues. Reviewing a growing literature (see also work reviewed in Smith 1989, 1990) these authors question the extent to which housing need is related to health problems and point to the difficulties of weighting medical needs against other priority claims. They show that systems of awarding medical priority vary considerably between local authorities and that there is little consistency in the decisions made by the various health professionals involved in medical assessments. Along with other public health physicians such as Parsons (1987) and Gray (1990) these authors question the role and involvement of clinicians in housing management decisions. Clinicians, they argue, may have little grasp of the complexities and difficulties of housing allocation, and their work here could simply legitimize *ad hoc* housing management decisions and contribute to the medicalising housing need. For Connelly and Roderick, therefore, the most useful role for public health physicians to play in housing policy decisions is not by participating in casework but by assessing local needs, evaluating the full range of local health care provision, and linking housing managers into a wider health care network. Clinicians should, they argue, move from a housing management to a planning, co-ordinating and health advocacy role, promoting health for all at a time of increasing homelessness and in the light of the decreasing affordability of much of the nation's housing stock.

Whether or not these views are acceptable, justifiable, and feasible to the wider body of housing managers and public health physicians, it is obvious to many commentators that the principles underpinning the medical priority system are fundamentally challenged by changes in the size and quality of the council rented housing stock and by the changing nature of demand for that stock. One response to the increasing difficulty of supplying good quality general needs council housing to the full range of medical needs applicants has been the development of more specialized forms of housing provision targetted towards specific and limited client groups. The problems and advantages of this 'special needs' perspective have been considered elsewhere (Clapham and Smith 1990; Smith 1990a, b). The key point is that the housing field most often caters for 'special needs' by the provision of purpose-built, and therefore frequently segregated dwellings packaged with special forms of health care or social support. While such initiatives have no doubt benefited many individuals, and while they may, in the present fiscal climate, be one of the few ways of harnessing new resources into the housing system, Chapter 6 shows that they are by no means a sufficient route to achieving independent living opportunities for people with mobility difficulties. The arguments Jenny Morris uses to persuade us of the problems here could equally well be applied to the question of special versus mainstream services for people with mental health problems or learning difficulties.

Chapter 6 draws attention to the failure of policy makers to provide housing that is physically suited to the needs of people with mobility, stretching and reaching difficulties. Morris points out that disabled people who need support often have to make a stark choice between entering residential care or resigning themselves to dependency on family and friends. Neither of these fulfils the demand for integrated or independent living that is such a central part of the international civil rights movement of disabled people. Her central point is that 'For many disabled people, unwanted dependence on others would disappear overnight if they lived in a physical environment which did not handicap them'.

In discussing the barriers to independent living for disabled people, Morris is, like many other authors in this volume, suspicious of the divisions of the housing stock into general and special needs segments. She hints, in fact, that this division is itself instrumental in undermining the citizenship rights of people with health related housing needs. Her persuasive argument is that disability should not come at the cost of its incumbents' right to homes of their own, provided in the same way and with the same range of tenure and locational choice as is available to any other citizen. Her review of the policies of a sample of local authorities in England and Wales suggests that, at the moment, this welfare ideal is severely compromized.

The incomes of disabled people tend to be disproportionately low (a consequence of exclusion from or discrimination within the labour market), and the majority of affordable housing for this group is in the council rented sector. As access to this sector has become more difficult, disabled people have become more vulnerable to homelessness. Yet, the surveyed authorities rarely had well developed policies for tackling this. Even where local authorities had made important steps in housing provision for minority groups, singles and older people, they often failed to tackle the housing problems of people with mobility difficulties in any systematic way. In general, housing departments had disappointingly little information on housing demand from disabled people or on the housing needs of disabled people on any area by area basis. No accurate data were held on the actual or potential supply of adapted accommodation or on the general mobility characteristics of the local housing stock.

Perhaps the most fundamental problem identified by Morris—and one which has a more general bearing on the housing options for for people with health needs—was a tendency to marginalize disabled people in a way that undermined their access to homes through the mainstream allocations systems. At best they are restricted to purpose-built, segregated and sometimes stigmatized forms of accommodation and serviced with standardized packages of care, that may be helpful in some ways, but which can ignore many individual needs. This tension between the ideal of independent living in the mainstream housing stock and the development of special provision for those whose needs remain neglected by mainstream systems is taken up in Chapter 7, where Roz Pendlebury and Peter Molyneux give sensitive discussion of the complex issues surrounding housing provision for people with HIV and AIDS.

Pendlebury and Molyneux begin by documenting the general failure of mainstream housing services to develop procedures for accommodating people with HIV and AIDS. This chapter illuminates the problems that can arise where housing needs are defined by professional providers without adequate input from service consumers. The authors aim to redress this imbalance by offering people with HIV and AIDS a forum for their views. They report on a pilot study of the satisfaction of tenants of special schemes and of the housing preferences of people with HIV and AIDS in south London. This study exposed high levels of dissatisfaction among council tenants who had often been placed in 'difficult to let' estates, and had experienced problems with heating, security issues, and bathroom and laundry facilities. The majority felt their housing was harming their health and undermining their wellbeing: and most wished to move. There was a clear preference for mainstream over special provision, but concern that the mainstream services operate with stereotypical views of people with AIDS, linking the illness with judgements about morality, and aligning it with scales of respectability and opprobrium.

The chapter on HIV and AIDS exemplifies many of the problems which housing policy can create for people with medical needs. In a restructuring welfare state, strategies which single out certain groups as having special and pressing needs are required to lever more resources into the housing system. But the very singling out of groups for special attention can serve further to isolate them from mainstream housing services, thus working against the principle of providing housing and health care options that are integrative and 'normalizing'. This tension between the need to harness resources at all (thus risking the stigma that can be attached to 'special' groups) and the ideal of channelling adequate servicing through mainstream provision, recurs time and time again in the housing for health literature.

The exercise of medical priority in the public sector, as discussed earlier, refers to the movement of people into dwellings that are 'healthier' for them. The development of special provision, outlined above, requires the development of new built forms and bundles of care. Chapters 8 and 9 look more explicitly at the link between these strategies, exploring the (generally understated) role of housing in the provision of community care. Although in the past housing has tended to be viewed crudely as the bricks and mortar element of care in the community, both papers argue that this understates the potential of the housing services generally, and of housing managers in particular. By taking this view, the authors both provide a critical assessment of the white paper on *Community Care*, and evaluate the ideals and ideas behind this legislation.

Paul Spicker's paper is concerned with the integration of accommodation, health care and social support for people whose needs most often qualify them for residential care. Residential care tends to be located at an extreme point on the 'special housing' scale: it is the setting in which particular client groups are housed together in order to receive a package of caring services tailored to their collective needs. Spicker argues that this polarization is unnecessary, but is encouraged by current approaches to community care which are based on an artificial distinction between care in segregated residential settings and care in the community more broadly. The separation of residential care from community care produces, in Spicker's view, a wasteful division of health services into those aimed at the general population and those targeted towards special client groups. To avoid this distinction (which can be inflexible, stigmatizing, and insensitive to individual needs) Spicker advocates policies allowing some separation between the care element of residential care and the accommodation element. This separation would allow the two services to be provided and combined in a range of flexible and imaginative ways according to the variety of need which exists in the real world. It would ally policies for residential care more closely with policies for community care, and so offer a wider range of opportunities for independent and integrated living even for people needing high levels of health servicing and social support.

In Chapter 9 David Clapham takes these arguments one step further, arguing for the complete integration of community care policies into mainstream housing policies and procedures. Clapham is critical of the cursory and superficial way in which housing is addressed by policy makers as they seek to develop the new community care packages. He argues that the accommodation element in community care has been, at best, attached to the flag of the special housing movement and, at worst, ignored altogether. Certainly, it has not been built into the mainstream housing services. This, in Clapham's view, is a mistake which threatens the viability of the new procedures. The housing element in community care, he argues, is being concentrated into programmes which have relatively few resources; are narrowly targeted; and are secondary to (and usually undermined by) the aims of the main housing policies and programmes pursued by Government. Clapham goes on to propose an alternative approach, based on the principle of normalization. Such an approach would force those developing community care to be concerned with broader questions of housing subsidy and finance, tenure choice, and housing management more generally. Rather than viewing community care as a small addition to existing housing policy, this would build it into the principles which underpin the whole of housing policy, thus orienting it as much to the aims of social poli-cy as to the ideals of the competitive market place.

Homelessness as a barrier to health care

Section III addresses the range of housing options open to people with medical needs: it considers the achievements and limitations of the housing system in providing homes and access to health care for people with health problems. Section III goes on to confront the harsh reality that, for many people with health problems situated in an increasingly market oriented housing system, there simply is no satisfactory affordable accommodation.

The possibility that people with health problems may be denied entry to the mainstream housing stock, or forced to leave it, is considered in chapter four. As Smith (1990a) and Shanks and Smith (in press) show, people with medical needs are often dependent on the openness of the public sector (especially where health problems depress incomes and inflate expenditure) and on the proper coordination of housing provision with the process of deinstitutionalization. Where the system fails, sick people will be vulnerable to homelessness: and once people with medical needs lack a fixed address, not only do their health risks increase but their access to primary medical care (and thus to the National Health Services more generally) appears to decrease.

The risks associated with life on the streets are obvious and are manifest in the vulnerability of homeless people to musculoskeletal problems, leg ulcers, hypothermia and so on. Many also face high risks from infectious diseases through overcrowded hostels and shelters, and those seeking a local authority home face a range of problems (from fire hazard to mould and cold) when placed in temporary bed and breakfast accommodation. Yet, despite these risks GPs routinely fail to register homeless people or people in temporary accommodation on their practice lists, and most practices are too inflexible in their appointment systems and call-back services to respond to the immediate health care needs of those homeless people who do contact them. All the chapters in part III highlight the health hazards to which homeless people are exposed; document the problems homeless people face in securing adequate health care; and explore ways in which access to health services for people without a fixed address might be enhanced.

Some of the factors affecting the health profile of homeless people are outlined in Chapters 10 and 11. Nigel Shanks points out that homeless people are not an homogeneous group, and that the health problems and health care needs of women have been particularly underestimated. Homeless women tend to experience a higher than average incidence of complications during pregnancy; have above average rates of hospital admission during pregnancy; and have lower than average birthweight babies. Their problems arise both from the fact of homelessness (physical hardships as well as psychological strain) and from their limited access to medical care. These observations are confirmed by Jean Conway who, in Chapter 11 assesses the health problems faced by another relatively neglected group—homeless families in bed and breakfast accommodation.

Conway points out that despite the local authorities' increased use of bed and breakfast accommodation to house families for long periods of time while their statutory right to permanent rehousing is investigated, there are very few studies of the effects of this generally substandard accommodation on occupants' health. Drawing on her study of mothers and children in hotel accommodation in London, Manchester, and Southend, Conway draws attention to the cramped, overcrowded, infested, and unhygienic living conditions many have to tolerate. Stress and depression as well as poor physical health were common, and pregnant women as well as small children were particularly vulnerable to illness and disease. As Shanks also observed in his research, access to health care services for this group was very limited: few were registered with GPs and few received health visitors, so few babies were subject to developmental checks with low rates of vaccination and immunization.

Taking up some of the concerns raised in Chapters 10 and 11 the remaining papers concentrate their attentions on ways of extending the primary care services to different groups of homeless people. Again there is a tension between what might be termed special schemes (ie care targeted specifically and exclusively towards homeless people) and mainstream initiatives (designed to enhance homeless people's access to the regular primary care services). An example of a 'special' initiative is discussed by Simon Ramsden in Chapter 12. Ramsden emphasizes the diversity of the homeless populations and stresses the complexity of their health profiles. He points out, however, that they have one common factor which is that their pattern of health service use differs from that of more securely housed populations. Ramsden's argument for the importance of 'special' schemes (which, like Shanks, he would see simply as an adaptation of the relevant mainstream services) is that this different pattern of use has to be taken into account by service providers. To illustrate this, he reviews the work of the Great Chapel Street Medical Centre which was set up in 1977 for young homeless people, the Wytham Sick Bay, set up in 1984 in Maida Vale, and a mobile surgery developed in 1987 to service those living rough and having little contact with hostels and day centres.

Rick Stern and Barbara Stilwell emerged from their work on the Single Homeless Health Action Research project interested in initiatives like those discussed by Ramsden, but convinced that an entirely different approach to the health needs of homeless people is required. They find an irreconcilable gap between the perceptions of health professionals and the aspirations of homeless people concerning the role and availability of health services. Even definitions of what health care services are and should be were not shared. Homeless people defined health care as a set of practices which reach well beyond the confines of medical intervention, emphasizing the importance of incomes, rights, other welfare services and, crucially, housing, to the success of health care schemes. The implications of Stern and Stilwell's paper are that health care should be linked with housing and other care facilities, that service provision should be coupled with a broader understanding of what poor health and health improvements consist of, and that health care should include a commitment to social and economic change as well as to the welfare of individuals.

The balance between developing special schemes for homeless people, and developing policies to reorientate mainstream services to be sensitive to a wide range of needs, including those of homeless people is considered by Sandra Williams and Isobel Allen who evaluate a set of health initiatives for homeless people in London. These services aimed both to extend new forms of health care to homeless people and to encourage the greater integration of homeless people into the mainstream health services. More than any other chapter, this essay draws out the tensions among the various groups of health professionals, and between these professionals, their supporting voluntary workers, and client groups. The authors underline the need for a flexible and multidisciplinary approach to health care provision and they conclude that while special services are better than none at all, the most satisfactory solution is an integrated primary care network which is able to treat homeless people in the same way, and to the same standards, as those who are housed.

The papers collected in this volume illustrate the central importance of housing issues for public health policy. Housing opportunities vary systematically in quality, cost and availability, yet **where** people live affects the types of health hazard they are exposed to and it conditions their access to medical care and other welfare services. Housing (or the lack of it) can, on the one hand, expose people to health risks, and deny them access to medical care; but housing provision may, on the other hand, be used as a safety net for those whose market incomes are depressed by illness, or whose current housing circumstances are harmful to their health. Housing is the crucial mediator between incomes and health, between proverty and illness. More than ever before there is an urgent need to reappraise the steady divorce of housing provision from the aims of social policy, and to reconsider the extent to which housing policy, in addition to its role in environmental and economic management might also be viewed more explicitly as an instrument of health care.

References

Audit Commission 1986 *Managing crisis in council housing.* HMSO, London

Building Research Establishment 1986 Remedies for condensation and mould in traditional houses. Video, BRE

Carr-Hill R A, Maynard R, Slack R 1990 Morbidity variation and RAWP. *Journal of Epidemiology and Community Health* **44**: 271–273

Clapham D, Smith S J 1990 Housing and 'special needs'. *Policy and Politics* **18**: 193–206

Clapham D, Kemp P, Smith S J 1990 *Housing and social policy.* Macmillan, Basingstoke and London

Curtis S, Hyndman S 1989 The need for change in information, organisation and resources: a study of housing dampness and respiratory illness. *In* Martin C, McQueen D *Readings in the new public health,* Longman, Edinburgh, 203–213

Department of the Environment 1988 *English house condition survey 1986.* London, HMSO

Gray M 1990 Out of the nineties and into housing. *Public Health Physician* **1**: 5–6

Hyndman S J 1990 Housing dampness and health amongst British Bengalis in East London. *Social Science and Medicine* **30**: 131–141

MacIntyre S 1989 The role of health services in relation to inequalities in health in Europe. *In* Fox J Ed *Health inequalities in European countries.* Gower, Aldershot

Malpass P, Murie A 1987 *Housing policy and practice.* Macmillan, London

Martin C J, Platt S E, Hunt S M 1987 Housing conditions and ill health. *British Medical Journal* **294**: 1125–7

Niner P 1989 *Housing needs in the 1990's.* National Housing Forum, London

Parsons L 1987 Medical priority for rehousing. *Public Health* **101**: 435–41

Platt S D, Martin C J, Hunt S M, Lewis C W 1989 Damp housing, mould growth and symptomatic health state. *British Medical Journal* **298**: 1673–8

Secretaries of State for Health, Wales, Northen Ireland and Scotland 1989a *Working for patients* CM555 HMSO, London

Secretaries of State for Health, Wales, Northern Ireland and Scotland 1989b *Caring for people* CM 849 HMSO, London

Shanks N, Smith S J in press. Public policy and the health of homeless people. *Policy and Politics* forthcoming

Sheldrick B 1988 Campaigning for warmer houses at an affordable cost. *Radical Community Medicine* Spring 24–30

Smith S J 1989 Housing and health: a review and research agenda. *Discussion Paper* **27**. Centre for Housing Research, Glasgow University

Smith S J 1990a Health status and the housing system. *Social Science and Medicine* **31**: 753–62

Smith S J 1990b AIDS, housing and health. *British Medical Journal* **100**: 243–4

Strachan D P, Elton R A 1986 Respiratory morbidity in children and the home environment. *Family Practice* **3**: 137–42

Strachan D P, Sanders C H 1989 Damp housing and childhood asthma, respiratory effects of indoor air temperature and relative humidity. *Journal of Epidemiology and Community Health* **43**: 7–14

PART I
HOUSING AND
ACCESS
TO
HEALTH SERVICES

2 Residential location as a gateway to health care

Sarah Curtis

To set the scene for the analyses of housing for health included in this book, this chapter reviews the evidence for a link between where people live and what service they receive from the health care system. The availability and quality of health services for an individual can vary according to one's residential environment and location in a particular region or neighbourhood in Britain. The aim of this chapter is to review some of the main factors involved in this association between home location and health care, although to do justice to the topic would require a fuller account, as provided in texts on medical geography, eg Haynes (1987). The following discussion gives examples of the complex interaction of these factors, but does not attempt to describe overall availability and quality of health care for the population of different residential areas, since this would require a detailed analysis of particular localities.

The following sections discuss questions of resource allocation for health care, and outlines those aspects of the availability and quality of health care which are likely to vary for people in different residential locations. However, before embarking upon these, some general observations need to be made about the problems of assessing availability and quality of health care.

Assessment of social or spatial variations in the availability of services should be made with reference to variation in need for services. Since the 1970s the literature on health care has drawn readers attention to a pattern of health service provision described by Tudor-Hart (1971) as the 'inverse care law'. This is the observation that: areas where provision of health care seem to be of a relatively low level and quality are also areas which show high levels of morbidity and mortality suggesting high levels of need; while the better served areas using more resources seem to have generally healthier populations, presumably with lower needs. Powell (1990) has made a critical review of studies which have tried to test the 'inverse care law' in Britain. He concludes that the evidence in support of this 'law' is rather limited and restricted by the problems of measuring need, availability and quality of care.

It can be argued that studies of equity in health care should concentrate on the final outputs of health care (impact on population health) rather than on intermediate output measures of health care delivery. However, the measurement of such final outputs is very problematic. One well known attempt to assess health care outcomes in Britain focuses on the idea of 'avoidable mortality', Charlton et al (1983). This approach has shown that mortality from diseases amenable to medical intervention is variable across the country. The method is attractive and has been taken up in countries outside Britain because data are relatively easily available, and because the approach may give a clearer indication of the impact of health care than general mortality patterns. However, such information is difficult to obtain in a reliable form for small geographical areas, and the relationships between avoidable mortality and specific aspects of the functioning of health care systems remain unclear without further research, Humblet et al (1986). Similarly, while perinatal mortality is sometimes argued to be an indicator of the varying effectiveness of maternity health services in different parts of the country, it is necessary to take into account factors such as distribution of low birthweight and congenital abnormality before attributing the variation in mortality to quality of health care (Botting and Macfarlane 1990; Tarnow-Mordi et al 1990).

If we try to consider health care in terms of intermediate outputs such as service provision, one of the problems is the substitutability of different forms of health care. 'Health care' includes not only the medical care provided for in-patients and out-patients in hospitals, but also the 'primary' health services provided by health care professionals such as general practitioners (GPs), health visitors, and domiciliary nurses. Many of the services provided by local authorities also contribute to maintaining good health and caring for the sick, so that, for example, the activities of environmental health departments and social service departments are also relevant to the question of access to health care. The activities of the commercial and non profit making agencies also play a role. It is very difficult to draw a picture of the spatial variation in overall availability and accessibility of professional health care for particular areas because these different services may to some extent supplement or substitute for each other. Furthermore, the role of the informal sector is very important both in the care of sick people and in its effect on access to services (through support such as car share or dial-a-ride schemes, helpers who obtain prescribed medicines on behalf of sick people, etc). The following discussion, therefore, only gives a partial view because it concentrates solely on health services provided by health care professionals.

The scale of analysis is also important to studies of equity in health care provision. The patterns observed at the broad regional level may conceal intra-regional variations. The availability of health care may vary within regions for geographically defined populations living in different types of area (for example the situation in inner cities and remote rural areas is discussed below). Furthermore, accessibility also depends on social and economic factors which operate differently upon different individuals. So we must beware of making assumptions about individuals because of ecological relationships associated with the areas where they live. Some of the social factors discussed below help to explain these individual differences.

An assessment of the factors likely to affect future geographical variation in the provision of care in Britain is further complicated by the uncertainty surrounding the implementation of present government policy for health care, embodied in the new legislation which requires health service reforms and the reorganization of community care. Even now, it is very unclear how the changes about to be introduced will influence patterns of health care provision because the government policy statements (Great Britain Parliament 1989a,b) lack detail about how purchasers should assess the health care 'needs' of the populations for which they are responsible and how providers will respond to purchasers requirements in an internal market for health care services. Some of the implications of the changes which might be anticipated from this restructuring in the health service are considered below.

Allocation of resources for health care

One of the processes which influence the geography of availability of health care at the regional scale is the system for allocating resources in the National Health Service (NHS). This process was reviewed in the mid-1970s by the Resource Allocation Working Party (RAWP), which gave much weight in its report to evidence supporting an 'inverse care' phenomenon operating with respect to NHS funding (Noyce et al 1974; DHSS 1975). The North—South differential in mortality in Britain has been very persistent over time (Britton 1990) and is often cited as one of the factors contributing to the North–South divide in wellbeing and the quality of life (eg Howe 1986; Curtis and Mohan 1989). It is associated with a similar broad regional differential in morbidity and living conditions. In the RAWP report, the situation of Regional Health Authorities (RHAs) in the north of the country with high standardized mortality ratios and low ratios of health care expenditure to population, was contrasted with the situation in the 'Thames' Regions (London and the surrounding area) which spent more heavily and had comparatively lower mortality levels. The implication was that the region in which people lived would effect their access to National Health care in England and Wales. Such a situation seemed to run counter to the objectives of the NHS, which had been set up in 1948 to create a health care service which could be equally available to all in need of it, regardless of age, income or place of residence.

A revised system of revenue allocation for National Health Services to Regional Health Authorities (RHAs) recommended by RAWP was introduced in the mid 1970s. It used mortality as a surrogate measure of population need in a formula designed to shift resources towards those areas which were apparently under resourced in relation to their population needs. The general effect of the RAWP formula was therefore to constrain growth in the south east of England more than in the north and west of the country. A similar type of formula (SHARE) was also introduced for Scotland.

The RAWP formula was applied to the planning of revenue expenditure from 1976–89, and it certainly achieved a general shift in spending towards 'need' related target expenditure by RHAs over the period. The formula has thus had significant effects on the amounts of money RHAs and their constituent districts have had to spend on health care locally, especially in the London area which has experienced negative or zero growth in real income over much of the period. However, it is not clear whether it also achieved greater equity of provision and access to health care in different parts of the country. This resource allocation system was implemented in a period of general retrenchment in public health care expenditure and at a time when health policies required general reduction of numbers of hospital in-patient beds in an attempt to shift more resources towards the out-patient and community care sector. These objectives may have interfered with the aim of greater equity in hospital care provision because when the 'resource cake' is shrinking it is more difficult to achieve greater equity in the size and quality of the slices being shared out. Moreover, the allocation of regional budgets was not accompanied by direct central control over the activities of local health authorities, so that there was a good deal of scope for variation in the interpretation of local need for services of different types. Furthermore, implementation of the RAWP recommendations did not affect expenditure on general practitioners' services provided under the NHS, although this spending may be contributing to geographical inequity in resource allocation (Bevan and Charlton, 1987) nor upon private health care provision outside the NHS.

The RAWP formula was reviewed in the mid 1980s (DHSS 1988) and as part of the NHS reforms, new systems of allocation of resources to RHAs have been introduced. For the 1990–91 financial year, these include a revised RAWP formula using a modified measure of need, effectively giving less weight to regional mortality differentials. In subsequent years the RAWP system will be abandoned altogether and the resource allocation formula will be essentially a form of weighted capitation payment, based on population numbers and demographic structure. Some allowance will be made for needs of District Health Authorities (DHAs) but the details of this weighting mechanism are as yet unclear.

District Health Authorities will become budget holders responsible for purchasing health care for their local population. The role of provision of health care will be split from this purchasing role, and in future, various partners in the public, private and voluntary sector will be involved in the provision of NHS health care. The availability and quality of care for the population of a district will depend heavily on the success with which the DHA management carries out this purchasing role, assessing the needs of the population and drawing up contracts with providers to meet these needs. It is necessary to include specification of quality as well as quantity and price of health care in contracts, and this is a major challenge to health authorities, who urgently need more information on the present and future requirements of their population.

Some DHAs are concerned that the estimates of numbers of people living in their areas may be too inaccurate to allow for proper estimation of their resource needs. They fear that they will not therefore be adequately resourced under the new system to provide for the local population. This is particularly likely for inner city DHAs with highly mobile populations, or with large ethnic minority populations and large numbers of homeless people and travellers, since these are all groups which are known to be under-enumerated in the population census. Areas prone to receive sudden influxes of migrants and refugees will also find it difficult to make accurate predictions of their needs. In London, Hackney's recent experience of arrival of Kurdish refugees and the current movement of Somali refugees into Tower Hamlets illustrate this type of problem. In rapidly growing suburban areas, population estimates between censuses seem likely to become progressively more unreliable as time elapses after the enumeration.

Provision of community health care

Having reviewed the impact of the system of resource allocation to RHAs, this discussion now moves on to consider the operation of services on the ground and how this varies from one area to another. The focus here is on some of the more local factors affecting provision of and access to care. It is often argued that primary health care, when combined with improved public hygiene measures and living conditions, has more effect on the health of a population than the availability of curative services provided in hospitals (McKeown 1979). I shall therefore start with discussion of these. Primary health care is provided outside hospitals by community health service professionals, including preventive services and health promotion. It is a major plank of the WHO *Strategy of Health for All* to develop and improve primary health care. In many countries it is argued that this could be achieved by shifting resources away from hospital treatment and towards the primary care sector. British health care policy stresses the need to develop care in the community rather than in institutions for people who are chronically ill or are recovering from illness (DHSS 1981). This policy also calls for good community health services if it is to be implemented effectively.

Community health care is provided in Britain by a number of health professionals, including general practitioners (GPs) and health visitors, domiciliary and practice nurses, health promotion officers, dental practitioners, and ophthalmic opticians. The remuneration of general practitioners, dentists, and opticians is administered centrally by the Medical Practitioners Committee, and locally through Family Health Service Authorities (FHSAs). They also have a role to play in monitoring the services and ensuring that they are adequately accessible for local populations. District Health Authorities at present provide community nursing and health visiting services, as well as other community health care in the fields of chiropody, psychiatry, physiotherapy, etc. The policies and performance of these authorities, the resources which they receive to provide services, as well as the practice of the health professionals themselves, are therefore important to the local availability and quality of community health care.

The implementation of community care strategies also requires adequate and appropriate housing for chronically ill people. For example it is impossible to ensure care in the community for a mentally ill person who is not provided with a reasonable standard of accommodation; also domiciliary support for a dependent elderly person is more feasible in suitably designed and equipped accommodation. Housing may be an important factor in the costs of caring (Equal Opportunities Commission 1982) and if suitable informal care cannot be provided to a dependent person living in their own home, or in their carer's home, then sheltered housing may be considered as an alternative to institutional care. There is a continuing shortfall of sheltered housing and housing suited to the needs of chronically disabled people (Butler et al 1983). In the past the private housing market had shown little interest in contributing to our stock of this type of housing although recently, this situation has begun to change. Williams' (1989) examination of the development of the private sheltered housing market provides an example of geographical variation in the operation of the private market, which is one of the factors likely to determine the type and quality of non-institutional care which can be provided at home to chronically ill people.

Access to general practitioner services

General practitioners are key actors in the provision of primary care. They also have an important effect on access to, and use of, hospital services considered below. In order to have the full benefit of GP services under the National Health Service, a patient needs to be registered with a GP. Variations in registration rates among the population therefore have implications for access to care. Clearly for those who are homeless or with no fixed address, this problem is most severe. The problems of access to primary care for homeless people is dealt with in more detail in later chapters of this book. Even for those who have a home, however, non-registration can present a problem. It is generally held that registration rates are lowest in areas of high population mobility, especially in inner urban areas of our major cities. A household survey was conducted by the OPCS in 1981 to examine the levels and reasons for non-registration prevalent in ten inner London boroughs (Bone 1984) and the results were compared with those from an earlier study of access to primary care in England as a whole (Ritchie et al 1981). The surveys showed that while about 1 per cent of the English population as a whole was unregistered, the proportion in inner London was 4 per cent, with a further 1 per cent of the London population registered only temporarily. The inner London survey showed that about half of those who were unregistered under the NHS had other arrangements for access to a GP and 38 per cent were attached to a doctor's private practice. Among those who were not registered, about 10 per cent had tried to get onto the NHS list of a GP but had failed to do so. Another 9 per cent had not tried because they thought that they might be ineligible, that it would be difficult to register, or they did not know how to do so. Altogether about 1 per cent of the inner

London population represented by the survey were unregistered although they wished to be so.

Data from the two OPCS surveys also showed that in inner London and in England as a whole, 7–8 per cent of the population had failed to register with the first doctor approached, usually because the doctor would not accept them. Generally the reason given by the doctor is that the practice list is 'full' and that no more patients can be accepted. Some doctors also try to limit their practice populations to residential areas close to their practice and will not accept patients living too far away. This has implications for access to a GP's care, since although, in principle, people are free to register with a doctor of their choice, in practice a minority of patients must apparently accept a practice which is not their first choice. Even more worrying was the evidence from the OPCS study in inner London that people with chronic illnesses and older people (who are likely to require more time than average from a GP) were more likely to have difficulties finding a doctor to take them. Among those over 60 years of age who tried to register with a doctor, 15 per cent were rejected by the first doctor they approached. For those under 60 the proportion was only 1 per cent.

Another disturbing aspect of the report was the widespread ignorance about the role of the Family Practitioner Committees (now renamed the Family Health Service Authorities) in helping patients to register. Only 7 per cent of the inner London survey respondents knew that the FPCs could arrange registration and very few had sought their advice.

Bone (1984) suggested that in inner London, but not elsewhere, problems of registration were becoming more common. There is speculation that they may be further aggravated by the new system of remuneration of GPs under the NHS reforms. It is argued that, under the General Practice Funding Scheme, large practices (which can become 'budget holders', managing a fixed sum of resources to care for their NHS patients) will have a financial disincentive to take on patients who will be 'expensive' to the practice because they have chronic illnesses. Some individual cases highlighted in the press have provided anecdotal evidence that this may indeed be happening, but systematic information is not available.

A good deal of attention has been focussed on questions of access to a GP in British cities, partly because the criteria used to assess the provision of GPs in different areas were thought to underestimate problems of access in such areas. In one of the studies which is often cited in support of the 'inverse care law', Knox (1978) examined physical access to GPs in four Scottish cities, and concluded that physical access to family doctors was inversely related to the spatial pattern of social deprivation in Aberdeen, Dundee and Edinburgh, although in Glasgow the pattern was more complex.

The Medical Practice Committee is unable to direct GPs to practice in particular areas because family doctors are contractors to the NHS, rather than employees. However, incentives are offered to doctors to work in 'designated' areas, considered to be 'under-doctored', while in other, 'restricted' areas, where provision is considered above average, entry of new doctors is restricted. Until recently, this classification of 'designated' and 'restricted' areas for GP provision depended on the average list size of practices in each medical practice area (small administrative units used by the Family Health Service). Several commentators (eg Butler and Knight 1975; DHSS 1979) criticised the system, partly because the criterion of list size did not adequately reflect need in different populations, and also because the medical practice areas were in some cases quite large and diverse, so that they were inappropriate units for defining local need.

Furthermore, restrictions and incentives did not seem very effective in directing GP movements; 45 per cent of new GPs positions in 1973 were in 'restricted' areas. This system has therefore given way to a more flexible system of additional remuneration for GPs practising in areas where the workload of doctors is likely to be relatively high. Several different indicators of varying need for a doctor's care in local populations have been proposed (Thunhurst 1985). One which has been widely adopted is the Under Privileged Areas Index (Jarman 1983), which combines census data on a range of socioeconomic indicators, including measures of overcrowding and residential mobility, seen by doctors as likely to be associated with higher workloads in deprived areas. The index typically points to higher needs in deprived inner city areas, and is used to calculate GP deprivation payments, allocating extra funds to GPs in respect of underprivileged populations living in their practice areas (Delamonthe 1990).

However, problems of access to general practice also exist in other types of area apart from the inner city. Remote rural areas, for example, typically have poor access to services in general, including GPs surgeries, although in terms of size of practice, rural areas seem quite well served. (Average rural list sizes remained slightly lower, at 1,970, compared with 2,042 nationally. Average list size fell by 13 per cent 1976–86 in medical practice areas classified as rural, in line with the national trend towards smaller list sizes (DHSS, 1988; table 3.26.) In rural areas, people will often have little choice of doctor since there may be only one practice operating in their area. Studies by authors such as Haynes and Bentham (1982) and Philips (1979) have shown that for rural populations with lower personal mobility (especially women with young families, elderly people, and people in less privileged socio-economic groups) branch surgeries are often a particularly important point of access to the doctor. Questions of quality of GP care available in these facilities are addressed below. The trend towards increasing size of practice and increasing concentration of practices into central, purpose built premises during the 1970s led to a reduction of branch surgeries and single practitioner facilities (for example, Norfolk lost 61 surgeries 1950–80 and the number of single handed practices fell by 57 per cent 1969–78 (Packman 1987). Clark and Woollett (1990) suggest that this trend has slowed or reversed in the 1980s although some areas, such as Dorset continued to lose village surgeries up to 1988. The growth of larger practices in rural areas may have implications for the amount of choice which patients can realistically exercize over the practice with which they are registered. In some cases there will be only one practice operating in the area.

The number of doctors operating rural practices is indicated by payments of rural practice allowances. Nationally the numbers of doctors receiving these payments has increased by 42 per cent between 1978 and 1987 and 28 per cent of all doctors received these payments in 1987 (Clark and Woollett 1990). However, it is not clear that this represents a disproportionate shift of general practice towards rural areas. The last two decades have seen a shift of population towards rural areas, especially in areas within reach of urban employment centres. Many doctors still receiving rural practice allowances may now be working in suburban rather than deeply rural areas, and the areas showing the greatest increases in rural practice payments are in the home counties and Gloucestershire, rather than more remote rural areas such as Norfolk, Wiltshire, Shropshire.

Family doctors in rural areas also play an important role in the dispensing of medical prescriptions in areas not served by pharmacies. Doctors may dispense medicines to populations living more than a mile from a pharmacy. Perversely, this arrangement may make the supply of dispensing services more precarious in some rural areas, because if a doctor opted to dispense medicines, a pharmacy could suddenly lose customers from its wider catchment area and become economically unviable. The Rural Dispensing Committee was set up in 1983 to arbitrate between dispensing doctors and rural pharmacies who might be serving similar populations. Several studies have underlined the importance of catchment population size for the operation of pharmacies. Knox (1981) has analysed the distribution of pharma-cies in Scotland in relation to population change, showing a posi-tive correlation between population growth 1950–80 and change in pharmacies in administrative areas. The general decline in numbers of pharmacies observed in the 1970s has apparently been halted, especially in rural areas with growing populations, but it remains the case that there are few pharmacies in villages of less than 1,000 people and villages of less than 3,000 people are more likely than not to be without a pharmacy (Clark and Woollett 1990).

Supply of community health services

Other types of community health service also show variations in the level of provision from one part of the country to another. For example, the ratio of population to dental practitioners shows marked regional and local variations. In 1985 the ratio ranged from 2,281 per practitioner in North West Thames RHA to 4,402 in Trent RHA. For both dental practitioners and family doctors one of the most powerful factors influencing practice location is the location of the medical school in which they are trained (Thexton and McGarrick 1983; Butler and Knight 1975). Areas close to medical schools, especially around London are likely to be better provided than average in terms of numbers of practitioners.

Several studies (Carmichael 1983; Todd and Walker 1980; OPCS 1985) have shown that in areas where the supply of dentists is less generous, population dental health is poorer (as measured in terms such as proportions who are adentulous, or by fillings: extractions ratio). However, within regions the less privileged social groups systematically show poorer dental health and lower use of dental checks and treatment. Here again, we find evidence that the impact of differential access on use of care is mediated by individual factors such as social class.

The provision of community nursing services also shows variations between different parts of the country (DOH 1989). Haynes (1987) discusses a study by Dunnell and Dobbs (1982) of community nursing in a sample of health districts in England and Wales which examined differences in the numbers of nursing staff employed, in relation to the numbers of children and elderly in the population, and in the amount of time spent per week caring for children and adults aged over 65 years. These differences did not show any systematic relationship with area characteristics, however, and there was no evidence that in rural areas community nurses spent more time than average travelling to patients' homes. In a study of DHAs in London, Powell (1986) examined a range of measures of primary care provision, including indicators of health visiting and community nursing activity. These measures show considerable variations in provision and activity levels, but overall his results showed equivocal evidence of the 'inverse care law', since many of the provision indicators were positively associated with measures of need in the population.

It does appear however, that in Inner London, difficulties of recruiting and retaining nursing staff can affect the cost of staffing significantly. This is true for nursing in general (Mohan 1988b), community nursing, and health visiting. One of the important factors in areas like London is the high living costs in relation to nurses' salaries (Buchan 1990). Housing costs are an important element in living costs, so that the housing market, compounded with a less attractive living and working environment, contributes directly to deficient supplies of staff for community services.

Quality of community health care

In addition to questions of access to health care, there is a related issue of the quality of community health services. Some studies have documented evidence that the quality of services received by people living in some parts of the country may be below the average for the country as a whole. One of the types of area highlighted by these concerns are inner city areas. At the beginning of the 1980s a report by the London Health Planning Consortium (1981) emphasized problems of poor quality of community care in Inner London, especially in general practice. Although list sizes are on average rather low in inner London, it was noted that an above average proportion of practitioners were elderly, single-handed and that many were working in poorly equipped practice premises. There was also a problem of access to a GP out of surgery hours because many used automatic answering machines to direct patients to deputising services. It was suggested that this was another example of the inverse care law operating in inner city areas which have been shown in many studies to have relatively high levels of morbidity and health care need compared with more privileged suburban areas (eg Curtis 1987b; Leavey 1982). Powell (1990) also suggests that the quality of general practice may on average be poorer in areas of high need for care.

The concern engendered by this report led to a study in Manchester which sought to establish whether problems in inner city general practice were to be found outside London. The results suggested that the problems were not more serious in inner Manchester than in the outer urban area and it was concluded that London might have rather specific problems (Woods 1983). A population survey in inner and outer city areas of east London also indicated that there was not strong evidence of greater dissatisfaction with GP services in the inner city area. While differences in expectations and propensity to express dissatisfaction might partly account for the latter findings, it does seem likely that patients assess the quality of general practice largely in terms of the rapport and approachability of their doctor, and that some of the other professionally defined criteria of quality of care (such as group practice, good practice equipment and efficient organisation of appointments) were less important to patients (Curtis 1987a).

Further important factors affecting quality of care from the patient's point of view are particular requirements which certain patients may have. This is particularly important, for example, for ethnic minority groups, who may place high priority on having a doctor who is from the same cultural group, or for women who prefer a female doctor. Because of such differences in individual requirements of patients it is not easy to compare different locations in terms of appropriateness of care delivery.

It is probably an oversimplification to condemn general practice as a whole in inner London as poorer than average. A more accurate picture may be in terms of very variable quality, with some very progressive and committed practitioners providing very high quality care in well organised and well equipped premises, while at the other end of the scale, there undoubtedly still exist practices where the organisation and quality of family doctoring is below average standards. In view of the difficulties experienced by some people in registering with their preferred doctor, these variations in quality beg the important question of whether some groups of the population gain access to the better practices more easily than others.

Several reports have also highlighted problems of providing good community nursing services in inner city areas. In 1979, a working party on the primary health care team identified declining urban areas as problematic for provision of care. The working party reported that:

> The poor quality of the housing stock produces a working environment which both intensifies the difficulties of providing medical and particu-larly nursing care in the community, and tends to affect adversely the morale of staff working in such conditions (Standing Medical Advisory Committee 1979:44).

The Cumberlege report (DHSS 1986) focused on the need to organise community care on the basis of neighbourhoods in order to ensure more comprehensive cover by health visiting and district nursing services, especially in areas where general practices overlapped in geographical space. The report was influential in the decentralisation of service delivery in many DHAs, although implementation of locality based services has progressed at different rates around the country. As a result, the organization and delivery of community health services may vary within DHAs, depending on the operation of neighbourhood primary care teams.

In some deprived inner city areas conventional models of community nursing have been supplemented by more appropriate modes of service delivery. For example, in Tower Hamlets, socioeconomic deprivation is widespread and there are large numbers of people from ethnic minorities, so that new strategies for delivering health care are needed. In one example of such a strategy, local health professionals and community workers are collaborating to provide services in a 'health bus' which tours local housing estates, bringing health care and health promotion services closer to the doorstep for local people.

Inner city areas are not the only 'special' areas where local factors may result in below average quality of community care for some patients. General practitioners services available to rural dwellers may also be less than optimal. For example, Fearn et al (1984) showed that in rural Norfolk, older people, women, manual workers and those without a car included relatively high proportions of people who always used branch surgeries to consult a doctor. The authors point out that this type of surgery is often not purpose built and is commonly less well equipped than the main surgery premises—in particular branch surgeries lack facilities such as receptionists, clinical equipment or patients notes *in situ* Those using these facilities were having to balance problems of access to main surgeries against the drawbacks of using a poorer facility. In villages without a doctor's surgery of any kind, home visits were no more frequent than elsewhere, but telephone consultations were more common. While certainly more convenient, such consultations may be less satisfactory than face-to-face contact with the doctor.

Haynes (1987) reviews findings from studies in very isolated rural areas which show that access to primary health care is sometimes restricted to less qualified personnel. In the Outer Hebrides, for example, patients often relied on the district nurse as the first point of contact with primary health services, in cases which in other areas would be seen by a doctor. Although this practice at least ensures some trained health care, it cannot provide for an illness the same level of medical skill and expertise as would be expected from a doctor.

Provision of hospital beds and hospital admissions

Access to hospital care is probably the issue which attracts most public attention in debates over the health service. When assessing availability of hospital care one should be careful when interpreting provision levels across the country, as expressed in terms of units of a service per unit of population. The factors which confuse the

Table 2.1. *Data on regional variation in hospital provision and treatment in England 1975 and 1988*

Regional Health Authority	Available beds in hospitals*		In-patient cases treated*	
	in 1975	in 1987/88	in 1975	in 1987/88
Northern	8.7	7.3	110	150
Yorkshire	8.8	6.7	112	153
Trent	7.1	5.9	91	132
East Anglian	7.3	6.0	97	131
N.W. Thames	9.0	6.1	109	121
N.E. Thames	8.4	6.5	115	140
S.E. Thames	8.7	5.8	112	139
S.W. Thames	10.0	6.8	101	119
Wessex	7.5	5.3	100	134
Oxford	6.6	4.6	106	120
South Western	8.8	6.3	105	138
West Midlands	7.3	5.8	97	136
Mersey	9.4	6.9	107	144
North Western	7.9	6.8	111	162
England	8.3	6.3	107	140

Source: Department of Health, *Health and Personal Social Services Statistics* 1987, table 4.8; Department of Health, *Health and Personal Social Services Statistics* 1989, table 4.6
Information reproduced with permission of the Controller of Her Majesty's Stationery office

Note: * no. per 1,000 population
Activity and bed figures relate to region of treatment
Population figures relate to region of residence
Figures are rounded to nearest integer for in-patient cases

picture include variation in throughput of patients in different hospitals, substitution of services, and flows of patients.

Table 2.1 shows the regional differences in provision of hospital in-patient beds in 1975 and 1988. In spite of the effects of the RAWP formula on resource allocation (as discussed by Hancock in this volume) there are still geographical differences in bed provision. However, bed availability does not have a simple relationship to hospital use, since although numbers of hospital beds have been falling, the number of in-patient cases has increased. It has been argued, for example, that attempts to rationalize hospital in-patient activity in the London area have failed because although the numbers of beds have been cut, the throughput has increased (Kings Fund College 1988).

Availability of hospital beds, including intensive care provision and emergency care also varies due to seasonal and daily fluctuations in pressure on hospital beds. Policies of bed reduction in hospitals have produced a situation in which hospitals have little spare capacity. In the winter months when the incidence of serious illnesses such as respiratory and cardiovascular conditions increases, pressure on hospital beds can increase sharply, sometimes resulting in the need to postpone elective surgery or to discharge patients earlier than would otherwise have been the case.

There are also several substitution effects to take into account. For example, in response to policies of reduction of inpatient services, there has been an expansion of day hospital places which to some extent provides an alternative to inpatient care. The rate of day cases treated per 1,000 population have more than doubled in England since 1975 and stood at 18.6 per 1,000 in 1988 (DoH 1989).

Another 'substitution' factor complicating the picture of regional patterns of hospital provision is the rapid recent development of the private hospital sector, which shows a very distinct spatial polarization, and is highly concentrated in the south east of England (Mohan 1988a). Any gains in equity in regional provision in the NHS hospital sector achieved through the operation of RAWP have been severely eroded (if not outweighed) by the operation of the commercial health care market which enables more privileged patients in the south east with private health insurance to take advantage of a supply of private beds in and around London which is much more generous than in other areas.

Flows of patients between administrative areas also complicate the pattern of health care. This is particularly true for hospital provision. In some parts of the country (notably in the London area covered by the four 'Thames' RHAS) cross boundary flows can become significant at the regional scale and they have a profound effect on the pattern of provision at the local level (Brazier 1987).

There is considerable evidence that hospital admission rates vary from one part of the country to another. Haynes (1985) compared regional rates of admission for different illnesses, demonstrating a two or threefold difference between the highest and lowest rates for several types of condition. Within regions, DHAs show considerable variations. The highest levels are recorded in inner city authorities where the resident populations are socially and economically deprived. At the more local level of electoral wards, admission levels within one district can also vary significantly. The discussion so far has shown that a large range of supply and access factors are likely to be acting on rates of admission to hospital from different geographical areas, but the need element in the equation is also important.

Need for hospitalization varies with morbidity in the population, but we have little systematic information on the prevalence or incidence of morbidity in the population, especially for small geographical areas. The RAWP formula discussed above used standardised regional mortality ratios as indicators of need for health care. But hospitalisation also shows an association with other factors related to morbidity, such as demographic and socioeconomic differences between the populations of different areas. The General Household Survey (OPCS 1989) showed that the proportion of the British population who had been in-patients over the last year was greatest for children, women of child bearing age, and, particularly for people aged over 75 years. Areas with large populations of older people will therefore tend to have relatively high hospitalization rates. For certain types of hospital care, especially maternity facilities, need is highest in areas where there is a large proportion of women of child bearing age. Inner urban areas where the population is socially and economically deprived also have higher levels of hospitalization, even allowing for the fact that these areas typically have a high level of access to hospital beds (DHSS 1988). Data from bed censuses have shown that hospital beds contain a disproportionately high number of people from deprived neighbourhoods (eg Bates 1983).

It has often been argued that poor living conditions which may exacerbate illness and are unconducive to the treatment or recovery of a patient, cause higher rates of hospital admission or longer hospital stays for the population affected. For example, a recent Home Office report suggested that high admission rates among Bangladeshis living in Tower Hamlets were partly due to unhealthy housing conditions and uncertainty that treatment instructions would be followed at home (House of Commons 1986). Similarly a recent study in Queen Elizabeth Hospital, East London, concluded that high rates of admission of children to hospital were associated with social deprivation and living conditions (Carter et al 1990).

An important factor in the admission of patients to hospitals is the role of the GPs in referring patients. Apart from doctors' professional judgements about whether a patient needs hospital care, their referral behaviour might be expected to depend on a range of variables including the availability of hospital services in the local area; their knowledge of consultant specialists in different hospitals; the facilities for simple tests and surgery in their practice premises; and the pressures put upon them by their patients. Langan and colleagues (1990) carried out a survey among doctors in Kingston and Esher DHA, which asked them to indicate the importance of different factors for their choice of hospital for their patients. The doctors most often attributed importance to the waiting time for care at a hospital. However, Wilkin and Smith (1987) in a study in Manchester, found no evidence that referral rates among doctors were strongly linked to GP or patient characteristics, nor to proximity to a local hospital. Research is still going forward to try to document and explain varying referral rates in a more satisfactory way (Roland et al 1990).

It might be argued that waiting lists for hospital services are a good indicator of level of supply and availability for services in relation to demand for care. Waiting list data show considerable regional variation in the proportion of patients waiting more than a year for operations (from 38 per cent in North East Thames RHA, to under 20 per cent in the Northern, Trent and Mersey HAs). These should also be interpreted with care, however, since the quality of record keeping may account for some of the apparent geographical variation and it has even been suggested that waiting lists are manipulated by those rationing health services in order to strengthen the case for more NHS resources (or perhaps, more cynically, to generate demand for private health care as a means of queue jumping) (Williams 1990).

The problem of waiting lists for hospital places has attracted much public attention (College of Health 1985) and it is one of the aims of the NHS reforms to reduce waiting times for elective surgery. The White Paper *Working for Patients* (Great Britain Parliament 1989a), which set out the case for the NHS reforms, identifies the reduction of waiting times as an important objective. The paper argues that this could be achieved by operating an internal market in which health authorities would be able to take advantage of regional and local variations in bed availability to purchase hospital care for their patients which may be provided by hospitals outside the local area or the region.

This division of the role of purchaser and provider in the NHS will probably have the effect of increasing cross boundary flows of patient and will also make it possible for health authorities to arrange contracts with hospitals in the private sector to care for NHS patients. While a certain range of 'core' services (such as accident and emergency services, some general medicine and surgery, geriatric and psychiatric care) will be assured in each district for the local population, other services may become more polarised, clustering into those hospitals which are most successful in a competitive market. Even more than at present, patients may have to travel to other districts or regions for particular specialties. If such increased movements of patients occur, the question may arise of whether the movement of patients affects the acceptability of hospital services for them.

Quality of hospital care

The question of quality of hospital services is attracting increasing attention as medical audit becomes more important for quality assurance. Methods for monitoring patient satisfaction are also being used increasingly. More evidence is therefore becoming available on factors such as perioperative mortality (Buck et al 1987; Lunn and Devlin 1987) and patient satisfaction with the quality of care (Green 1989; Thompson 1988). However, while there are clearly important differences between hospitals, at this stage it is not possible to identify systematic geographical variations in these factors.

Variations in the age and design of hospitals can be significant for the quality of the care they provide. Typically, inner city hospitals are among the oldest in Britain, having been founded as charitable institutions over a century ago. Those long established teaching hospitals and centres of excellence in important specialties generally provide a high standard of care. However, in the more minor institutions it is difficult to maintain good standards because of spending cuts and outdated buildings and equipment. Davidson (1987) has graphically described these sorts of problems operating in an inner London hospital.

Close physical residential proximity to hospital care may not be very important to outcomes of most types of hospital services, but an obvious exception is the accident and emergency (A&E) services, for which time taken to reach the hospital can be critical. Since 1962, when the Platt Report (DHSS 1962) recommended rationalization of these services and concentration into larger and more fully equipped hospitals, the numbers of A&E facilities have declined. Haynes (1987) observes that in England and Wales, the number has fallen from 789 in 1962 to less than 200 in the 1980s, and that there are now large areas of Highland Scotland, the Scottish Borders, Central Wales and Devon and Cornwall which are more than 20 miles from an A&E facility. Clearly there is a fine balance to be resolved between the disadvantages of delay in obtaining emergency treatment because of these long travel times as against the benefits of more complete and sophisticated equipment and specialised staff in the major A&E centres.

The quality of A&E services in some areas is also affected by what is often referred to as 'inappropriate' use of casualty. This is most often reported in large cities, particularly London, where many patients present minor injuries and illnesses which might have been treated in a general practitioner's surgery. The phenomenon is usually taken to be a reflection of the inadequate access to good GP services in these areas as discussed above, particularly affecting people who are homeless or highly mobile. It might be argued that it would be better for hospitals to accept that this type of use will be made of their casualty units and make better provision for it. However, while this use of A&E is considered inappropriate, it tends to lead to overcrowded units with long waiting times, detracting from the quality of these services. Here again, a substitution effect is having an impact on the availability and quality of hospital services.

Conclusion: Area and individual factors in access to, and quality of, health care

The discussion above has demonstrated a range of service factors which may influence access to care and quality of care for users. In some cases these factors seem to be associated with particular types of area, such as inner cities or remote rural areas, which have received most attention in the literature. Historically, National Health Services have also been more generously funded in the south east of England than in the north and west, where mortality and morbidity indicators suggest that need for hospital care is greater. However, there are also more arbitrary differences between health authorities at the regional and district level, as well as growing variation within districts as decentralisation to neighbourhood level increases scope for local management and local initiatives. These differences reflect variations in policy and practice and often depend at the local level on the activities of individual health professionals. They are therefore difficult to summarize and hard to predict. The reforms proposed for the NHS seem likely to increase local variability in service provision partly because of the tendency for spatial polarization of services provided on free market principles.

Because demographic, socioeconomic and ethnic characteristics of local populations have profound implications for health status and service needs, it is difficult to make systematic comparisons between different areas of the country in terms of the match between provision and need. On the other hand, some studies have expressed concern that, at an aggregate level, an inverse care law may operate because shortcomings in service provision and quality are most serious in areas where need is most prevalent.

The inverse care law may also operate at the level of individuals. Another conclusion which emerges from many studies is that the individual characteristics of patients may make them particularly vulnerable to variations in accessibility and quality of services. Elderly people, women, ethnic minorities, and those who are without a car, who are not owner occupiers of their homes, or who have manual occupations are all groups of particular concern from this point of view, since they have health care needs which are often above average. While these groups are often the heaviest users of health services, there is continuing unease over whether the quantity and quality of services they use are proportionate to their greater than average need levels. These are groups which are often disadvantaged in terms of housing and other aspects of welfare, so that constraints on access to the best and most appropriate health care are likely to be compounding their disadvantage.

References

Bates T 1983 *Patient census study: social factor analysis report 1249. North East Thames Regional Health Authority Management Services,* London

Bevan G, Charlton J 1987 Making access to health care more equal: the role of the general medical services *British Medical Journal* 26 Sept, **295**: 764–67

Brazier J 1987 Accounting for cross boundary flows *British Medical Journal* 10th Oct, **295**: 898–900

Bone M 1984 *Registration with general medical practitioners in inner London.* HMSO, London

Botting B, Macfarlane A 1985 Geographic variation in infant mortality in relation to birthweight 1983–85: chapter 5 pp 47–56 in Britton, M. *Mortality and geography: A review in the mid-1980s.* HMSO, London

Britton M (Ed) 1990 *Mortality and geography: a review in the mid 1980's, England and Wales, OPCS Series DS9.* HMSO, London

Buchan J 1990 Keeping nurses mobile. *Health Service Journal* 15 March, **1592**: 396–97

Buck N, Devlin H, Lunn J 1987 *The report of the confidential enquiry into perioperative deaths. King's Fund,* London

Butler A, Oldman C, Greve J 1983 *Sheltered housing for the elderly: policy, practice and the consumer.* Allen and Unwin, London

Butler J, Knight R 1975 The choice of practice location. *Journal of the Royal College General Practitioners* **25**: 496–504

Carmichael C 1983 General dental service care in the northern region. *British Dental Journal* **154**: 337–39

Carter F et al 1990 Material deprivation and its association with childhood hospital admission in the East End of London *Maternal and Child Health* 15 (6): 183–7

Charlton J, Hartley R, Silver R, Holland W 1983 Geographical variation in mortality from conditions amenable to medical intervention in England and Wales Lancet 26th March, 691–96

Clark D, Woollett A 1990 *English village services in the eighties* Rural Development Commission, London

College of Health 1985 *Guide to hospital waiting lists.* College of Health, London

Curtis S 1987a The patient's view of general practice in an urban area. *Family Practice* **4** (3):200–6

Curtis S 1987b Self reported morbidity in London and Manchester: intra-urban and inter-urban variations. *Social Indicators Research* **19**: 255–72

Curtis S, Mohan J 1989 The geography of ill-health and health care in Lewis J. and Townsend A (eds) *The north south divide*. Paul Chapman, London, 175–191

Davidson N 1987 *A question of care: the changing face of the National Health Service*. Michael Joseph, London

Delamonthe T 1990 Deprived area payments *British Medical Journal* **300**:1509–10

DHSS 1962 *Report of a sub-committee on accident and emergency services*. HMSO, London

DHSS 1975 *Sharing resources for health in England and Wales*. HMSO, London

DHSS 1979 *Patients first*. HMSO, London

DHSS 1981 *Community care*. HMSO, London

DHSS 1986 *Neighbourhood nursing: A focus for care* HMSO, London

DHSS 1988 *Review of RAWP*. DHSS, London

DoH (Department of Health) 1989 *Personal health and social services statistics 1989 edition*. HMSO, London

Dunnell K, Dobbs J 1982 *Nurses working in the community*. HMSO, London

Equal Opportunities Commission 1982 *Who cares for the carers? Opportunities for those caring for the elderly and handicapped* Equal Opportunities Commission, London

Fearn R, Haynes R, Bentham C 1984 Role of branch surgeries in a rural area. *Journal of the Royal College of General Practitioners* **34**: 488–91

Great Britain Parliament 1989a *Working for patients, Cm555*. HMSO, London

Great Britain Parliament 1989b *Caring for people: community care in the new decade and beyond, Cm 849* HMSO, London

Green J, 1989 On the receiving end. *Health Service Journal* 15th June: 728–29

Haynes R 1985 Regional anomalies in hospital bed use in England and Wales. *Regional Studies* **19**: 19–27

Haynes R 1987 *The geography of health services in Britain*. Croom Helm. London

Haynes R, Bentham, C. 1982 The effects of accessibility on general practitioner attendances and inpatient admissions in Norfolk, England. *Social Science and Medicine* **16**: 561–64

Howe M 1986 Does it matter where I live? *Transactions, Institute of British Geographers* **11**(4):387–410

House of Commons 1986 *First report of the Home Affairs Committee, Session 1986–87: Bangladeshis in Britain Volume 1*. HMSO, London

Humblet P, Lagasse R, Moens G, Van de Voorde H, 1986 *Atlas de la mortalite evitable en Belgique 1974–78. Ecole de Sante Publique*, Universite Libre de Bruxelles, Brussels

Jarman B 1983 Identification of underpriveleged areas. *British Medical Journal* **286**: 1705–8

Kings Fund College 1988 *Back to back planning.* King's Fund. London

Knox P 1978 The intra-urban ecology of primary health care: patterns of accessibility and their policy implications *Environment and Planning A,* **10**: 415–35

Knox P 1979 Medical deprivation, area deprivation and public policy *Social Science and Medicine* **13D**: 111–21

Knox P 1981 Retail geography and social wellbeing: distribution of pharmacies in Scotland. Geoforum **12**: 225–264

Langan J, Stephenson A, Cochrane D 1990 How big can we grow? *Health Service Journal,* 6th Sept: 1320–21

Leavey R 1982 *Inequalities in urban primary care: use and acceptability of GP services.* Department of General Practice, DHSS Research Unit, University of Manchester, Manchester

London Health Planning Consortium 1981 *Primary health care in inner London.* DHSS, London

Lunn J, Devlin H 1987 Lessons from the confidential enquiry into perioperative deaths in three NHS regions. *Lancet* 12th December: 1384–86

Mckeown T 1979 *The role of medicine.* Blackwell, Oxford

Mohan J 1988a Restructuring privatisation and the geography of health care in England 1983–87. *Transactions Institute of British Geographers* **13**: 449–65

Mohan J 1988b Spatial aspects of employment change in Britain: I : aggregate trends. *Environment and Planning* **A 10**: 7–23

Moore A, Roland M 1989 How much variation in referral rates among GPs is due to chance? *British Medical Journal* **298**: 500–2

Noyce J, Snaith A, Trickey A 1974 Regional variations in the allocation of resources to community health services. *Lancet* **7857**: 554–57

OPCS 1985 *General household survey 1983.* HMSO, London

OPCS 1989 *General household survey 1986.* HMSO, London

Packman J 1987 *Rural disadvantage and service loss in Norfolk.* Norfolk Rural Community Council, Norfolk

Phillips D 1979 Spatial variations in attendance at general practitioner services. *Social Science and Medicine* **13D**: 169–181

Powell M 1986 Territorial justice and primary health care: an example from London. *Social Science and Medicine* **23**: 1093–1103

Powell M 1990 Need and provision in the National Health Service: an inverse care law? *Policy and Politics* **18(1)**:31–7

Ritchie J Jacoby A Bone M 1981 *Access to primary health care.* HMSO London

Roland 1990 Understanding hospital referral rates: a user's guide. *British Medical Journal* **301**: 98–102

Standing Medical Advisory Committee 1979 *The primary health care team: report of a joint working group of the Standing Medical Advisory Committee and the Standing Nursing and Midwifery Advisory Committee.* DHSS, London

Tarnow-Mordi, W et al 1990 Predicting death from initial disease severity in very low birthweight infants: a method for comparing the performance of neonatal units *British Medical Journal* **300**: 1611–14

Thexton A, McGarrick J 1983 The geographical distribution of recently qualified dental graduates, 1975–80 in England and Wales *British Dental Journal* **154**: 71–6

Thompson A. 1988 The practical implications of patient satisfaction research. *Health Service Management Research* **1 (2)**; 112–19

Thunhurst C 1985 The analysis of small area statistics in planning for health. *Statistician* **34**: 93–106

Todd J, Walker A 1980 *Adult dental health, England and Wales, 1968–78, OPCS.* HMSO, London

Tudor-Hart J. 1971 The inverse care law. *Lancet* **1971(i)**:405

Wilkin D, Smith A 1987 Variation in general practitioner's referral rates to consultants. *Journal, Royal College of General Practitioners* **37**: 350–353

Williams A 1990 Escape the trap. *Health Service Journal* 15th Feb:242–43

Williams G 1989 Speculative house building and new housing markets; the role of private sheltered housing. *Planner* **75 15**: 16–20

Woods J 1983 Are the problems of primary care in inner cities fact or fiction? *British Medical Journal* **286**: 1109–12

3 Housing conditions, health needs and the use of hospital services

Karen Hancock

Introduction

The purpose of this paper is to show how the use of National Health Service (NHS) hospital services is linked to housing conditions, and other social factors, and to postulate some plausible causal mechanisms. A main concern is to show that in spite of the recognition by Smith (1989) of an increasing de *jure* separation between health policy and housing policy at governmental level, there have been some de *facto* links between them. This paper is not directly concerned with the impact of housing conditions on health status, although this has a bearing on the theory outlined here; nor does it explicitly investigate the effects of health status on housing consumption opportunities. The concern is rather to examine the pattern of consumption of hospital resources in the NHS to determine what factors the system itself uses to allocate resources to patients.

The analysis shows that the factors which are used to indicate need for hospital resources at lower levels of the hospital service are not always strictly medical, and, more importantly, not the same as the factors which govern, the way in which NHS resources are allocated at higher levels. However, recent proposed policy changes in the White Paper *Working for Patients* (HMSO 1989) will have the effect of modifying the national level resource allocation formula so as to bring it more into line with the pattern of resource use at lower levels. In consequence, the resource allocation system of the NHS seems poised to become more explicitly responsive to local housing and social conditions.

The paper is organised as follows: the first section is devoted to outlining the theory of the ways in which housing conditions, health needs and use of hospital resources might be linked under the NHS — a system which employs non-market modes of resource allocation. Next follows a description of the data used to examine these hypotheses and an outline of the key results. A final section concludes with a discussion of policy implications.

Determinants of the use of hospital services

The NHS was brought into being at least partly to avoid the inequalities of a market insurance-based health care provision system in which treatment depended both on morbidity and on ability to pay. At the national level, the determinant of national average use of hospital services is Government policy, because it is Government policy which explicitly decides the total NHS budget. It is also Government policy which determines the allocation of the NHS Hospital and Community Health Services (HCHS) budget to the fourteen English Regional Health Authorities. The HCHS budget is divided among the Regions according to the RAWP formula[1]. The objective of this resource allocation formula is to provide equal access to health care to those in equal need. The Government's view of the determinants of need for hospital resources may therefore be inferred from the formula. The principal indices of need for hospital resources in this formula are population, age and sex structure, and an index of mortality relative to the age and sex-specific national averages known as Standardized Mortality Ratio (SMR)[2].

The RHAs then divide up their budgets to the 192 District Health Authorities (DHAs) according to their own sub-regional formulae, although most regions simply replicate the RAWP formula to measure the DHA's relative needs for resources. Some RHAs have taken other factors such as 'social deprivation' into account.

Since there is no charge to the patient for the use of hospital facilities at the point of consumption there is, from an economist's perspective excess demand at zero price. The rationing of hospital facilities is therefore effectively carried out by GPs, who screen cases before referring them, as well as by consultants, who decide which cases to admit. When considering which cases to admit, and when to send patients home, these 'gatekeepers' will take into account several factors, such as the patient's medical need for hospital treatment, competing demands on the facilities arising from other patients, and to a certain extent, the patient's home conditions. At the individual level, therefore, the amount of hospital resources consumed by a member of a particular local population depends on what I have termed elsewhere the local 'supply regime' (Butts, Hancock and Swales 1989). The local supply regime is simply the prevailing local view of medical priorities or, put another way, the implied local rationing system. In part, the rationing system will depend on the total volume of resources relative to the demands upon them, but it will also depend on the ways in which those resources are allocated amongst competing users locally. The two main aspects of the research reported here attempt to determine, first, whether the needs indicators implicit in local supply regimes are consistent with those used in the national level formula and, second, whether there is consistency across space—in particular between regions— in the needs indicators used. But the main interest lies in the extent to which there is a relationship between factors such as patients' home conditions and hospital resource use: factors which were not taken into account in the original RAWP formula[3].

The Government element in the resource allocation process, ie, the RAWP formula, has been, as any method for allocating resources will be, the subject of much controversy. The debate is summarized by Mays (1987). Essentially, there are three main issues:

1   Is a measure of death rates (SMRs) an adequate proxy for morbidity?;
2   If so, what weight should it have in a needs formula?;
3   Is mortality the only relevant factor governing the need for hospital resources?

It is the third issue which is the primary concern of this essay. The other two issues are spelled out in more detail elsewhere (Butts, Hancock and Swales 1989). Briefly, however, the use of SMRs solely as a proxy for the excess morbidity, over and above a population's age and sex structure, has been questioned on a number of grounds. First, clearly there is a strong argument that sickness is not the same as death and that those who suffer from non-fatal illnesses can be heavy users of hospital resources. Because of this, some authors have argued that a vector of 'social factors', including housing conditions, are a better proxy for morbidity, especially sub-regionally. Second, relating resource allocation to a region's death rates might be argued to be erecting a totally inappropriate incentive structure for a health service! The question of the appropriate weight which SMRs should receive in a needs formula centres around whether there is any theoretical justification for the current value of one.

The third set of arguments concerns the point that a patient needs to be more than simply sick to consume hospital resources

45

and therefore morbidity proxies are by themselves inadequate to capture relative need for hospital resources. There can be a number of influences at work here. For example, it may be argued that in areas where there is low GP provision, patients might put more demand pressure on hospitals because less screening is carried out by GPs. In such areas, patients are more likely to present themselves at the local casualty department with health problems which might normally be treated in a GP's surgery. Since low GP provision is more often to be found in deprived, inner city areas, social deprivation might be a good predictor of this extra hospital demand. It is likely that homeless people, who often tend to bypass GPs, and present themselves directly to accident and emergency departments, are also concentrated in such deprived inner city areas.

There is another, more direct, link between social deprivation and need for hospital resources. It is more difficult for GPs to treat patients in their own homes if their home conditions are poor or if they have relatively little access to family support. *Ceteris paribus*, such patients are more likely to be admitted to hospital, and once admitted, they are, for the same reason, more likely to stay longer.

These arguments point to a difference between resource allocation decisions at a local level, and those made at a national level. In particular, they suggest that the pattern of *resource use*, as distinct from the resource allocation formula, could be influenced by the home and neighbourhood conditions of the patients. A more specific argument about the importance of social deprivation or home conditions on the amount of hospital resources consumed by the populations of small geographical areas may be made in the following way. The amount of hospital resources consumed by the population of a given geographical area is the product of the number of admissions from that population and the average length of stay in hospital in that area. Dealing first with the decision to admit a patient to hospital, the probability of a particular individual from that population being admitted to hospital can be conceived of as the outcome of a sequence of decisions. First, the patient feels ill, then he or she consults a GP. The GP may refer the patient to hospital, or the patient may self-refer through the A&E department. Whether the patient is admitted is dependent on whether a free bed exists. Each stage of this process is conditional upon the previous stage occurring and may thus be modelled as a set of conditional probabilities, since if any one of the following probabilities is zero, then no admission occurs:

1. P(admit) = P(feeling ill). P(consulting GP). P(hospital referral). P(a free bed exists)

Each of these probabilities is influenced by a different party's judgement about need: the individual, the GP and the consultant/hospital. Finally, the probability that a free bed exists is influenced by, among other factors, the existing pattern of resource allocation, ie, the RAWP formula. Given the previous discussion, the following hypotheses concerning the determinants of these probabilities seem reasonable.

2. P(individual feels sick) = f (death rates and/or social factors, age/sex)

In equation 2, death rates, age/sex and social factors are proxies for the morbidity of the population with respect to conditions leading to hospital admission. The probability that an individual feels sick is expected to be increasing in death rates, decreasing in social factors (if they are measured such that higher values means less social deprivation) and increasing in the proportions of the population which fall into the high user groups: generally the young, the elderly and women of childbearing age. It is worth noting that as well as poor home conditions giving rise to ill health directly (as discussed in Smith, 1989), it is also the case that home conditions are likely to be a proxy for wealth (consumption opportunities) and also preference patterns which may be determinants of health. For example, higher income groups have lower rates of cigarette smoking and a better diet.

3. P(consults GP) = g (social factors, GP provision)

The probability that an individual consults a GP, given that he or she is sick, is thought by some to be positively related to social factors, thus mitigating the hypothesized tendency for social factors to be inversely related to expressed demand for hospital resources. Of course, it has to be recognized that homeless persons rarely consult GPs at all and the normal method of admission is for them to present with acute problems at hospital A&E departments. In fact, this study, and arguably the RAWP formula, both in its original and in its modified form, take little account of homeless people and their health needs at all. Another hypothesis about the relationship between social deprivation and GP consultation rates concerns the suspicion that the middle classes are overrepresented for any given level of morbidity and age and sex structure.

4. P(referred to hospital) = h (social factors, GP provision)

Equation 4 expresses the view that the probability that a patient is referred to hospital, or self-refers, is related to social factors and to the volume of GP provision. The quality and nature of the patient's home background is likely to influence a GP's decision on whether a particular medical condition should be treated in hospital. For example, where a patient lives in poor accommodation, or lacks family support, the GP is more likely to admit the patient to hospital. Again, the level of GP provision might affect the rate of referrals. The relationship between GP provision and hospital referrals might be complementary to or substituting for the GP provision.

5. P(a free bed exists) = j (access)

Finally, the probability that a patient referred to hospital will gain admission to a hospital bed depends on what might be termed 'access'. Access might be considered to be a function both of the patient's distance from the hospital and of the relative scarcity of hospital beds. Distance is likely to be a factor in the accessibility of hospital beds because information transmitted through informal networks about the availability of more distant beds is likely to be less good than about those closer by. It may also be argued that patients prefer to be admitted to more easily accessible hospitals. The relative scarcity of hospital beds depends on the number of available beds and the volume of demands being placed upon them by the region's population. A measure of access was developed based on these principles. A more detailed explanation of its derivation may be found in Butts, Hancock and Swales (1989).

Many of the relationships expressed in equations 2, 3 and 4 have variables in common, and when it comes to statistical testing, the different effects will be inseparable. Thus, summarizing the elements of the above discussion into one equation, yields::

6. AM_i = f (age/sex, SMRs, GP provision, social deprivation, access)

where AM_i = hospital admissions per 1,000 population of geographical area i

The remaining component of the consumption of hospital resources by patients is the average length of stay in hospital. For much the same reasons as apply to admission decisions, it is hypothesised that decisions on length of stay depend on the age and sex structure of the population, the volume of GP provision, accessibility and a group of social factors, including the patient's home conditions. Therefore:

7. LOS_i = g (age/sex, GP provision, access, social factors)

where LOS_i = average length of stay in hospital of a patient resident in geographical area i. The total consumption of hospital resources by patients from a given geographical area, i, is the product of admissions per thousand (AM_i) and average length of stay (LOS_i). This gives a relationship for the consumption of bed-days per thousand population of geographical area i (BD_i) as follows:

8. BD_i = h (age/sex, SMRs, GP provision, access, social factors)

There is no theoretical justification for any particular functional form. However, given the nature of the admissions process outlined above, a multiplication form seems appropriate. However, because many of the social variables have possible zero values, they were included in the estimating equations in a linear, additive form. The estimating equation therefore took the specific form:

9. $\log (BD) = \alpha_0 + a_1\log(EBD) + \alpha_2\log(SMR) + \alpha_3\log(GPLIST)$
$+ \alpha_4\log(GPQUAL) + \alpha_5\log(ACCESS) + \Sigma\beta_jSF_j$

where EBD represents expected bed-days per 1,000 population, ie, the bed-days rate that would apply to geographical area j if the bed-days per thousand registered by each age and sex group were the same as the national average for each age and sex group; SMR represents the standardised mortality rate; GPLIST represents the size of GP patient lists; GPQUAL represents the average quality of GP provision in the area; ACCESS represents the access measure and SF_j represents social factor j.

In equation 9 the coefficients αj can be interpreted as elasticities. That is, the coefficient is a unit-free measure of the responsiveness of bed-days to a small change in the value of the relevant independent variable. The β_j can be interpreted as semielasticities, ie, as a measure of the proportionate change in bed-days per thousand when the independent variable increases by one. Because the social variables are expressed as percentages, this represents a particularly useful characteristic.

There are some differences of detail between equation 9 and the RAWP formula. In the RAWP formula, the SMR variables are medical condition-specific and weighted by the hospital costs for these conditions. This means that if a region were to have a high SMR in a condition which were particularly resource-intensive, then this would be indicative of a particularly high needs population. Condition-specific SMRs are not suitable for the level of geographical disaggregation at which this analysis is conducted. In addition, the SMR data which are used here are calculated for the population aged up to 75 years only. In the RAWP formula, all-age SMRs are used. The argument for using the SMR to age 75 is that areas with low full age range SMRs are likely to have higher

49

needs for care of the elderly (since more of their population sur-
vive to old age). It is this argument which has resulted in the
Scottish SHARE formula using SMRs only to age 65. In actual
fact, three forms of SMR (all-age, to age 75, and to age 65) were
calculated and tested out empirically. SMRs to age 75 consistently
gave the better results on statistical criteria. SMRs to age 75 are
simply an area's actual death rate divided by the death rate the
area would have had if each age and sex group up to age 75 in its
population had the corresponding national death rates.

Data

The empirical work described here attempts to account for the
pattern of the use of hospital resources between the populations
of small geographical areas within a unified supply regime, which
is taken at this stage to be a region. In principle, the smaller the
intraregional areas chosen as the units of observation the better:
the smaller the areas, the greater the number of observations per
region and the less likely that resource-use patterns will simply
replicate the formulae used by the regions to allocate resources to
districts. Electoral wards were selected as the greatest degree of
geographical disaggregation which was practical: greater disaggregation to the level of Census Enumeration Districts would have
generated data difficulties.

Six English RHAs provided data for this study: S E Thames, N
W Thames, Wessex, W Midlands, Trent and Mersey. These were
thought to be broadly representative of health authority regions in
England as a whole, but the principal criterion for inclusion in the
study was the availability of postcoded Hospital Activity Analysis
(HAA) data. However, there appeared to be problems with the
data from three of the regions and only results obtained from the
remaining three regions for which the data proved to be more reliable are reported here: S E Thames, Wessex and Trent[4]. In addition, certain electoral wards are excluded from the analyses. These
are: electoral wards with boundary changes since 1981; those
wards within districts having outflows of admissions to other
regions greater than an arbitrary 5 per cent of total admissions
and those wards within DHAs defined by the DHSS as 'Teaching
Districts'[5].

All the variables used in the regressions are listed and defined in
Table 3.1 It should be noted that population data for 1985 had to
be estimated by assuming that the rate of change of population of
an electoral ward equalled the rate of change for the district in
which it was located, since the Office of Population Censuses and
Surveys (OPCS) only provides district level population estimates.

Table 3.1. *Variable list*

BDAYS	Total bed-days per thousand of the electoral ward's population, 1985, for non-psychiatric,non-maternity admissions.
ACCESS	Computed access scores for electoral wards[6]
SMR75	Standardized mortality ratios up to age 75, averaged 1981–85
SPAR	% of households being single parent families, 1981
ELDAL	% of households consisting of lone elderly, 1981
MOVED	% of households having moved at least once within the previous 12 months, 1981
UNEMP	% of residents aged 18 and over seeking work or temporarily sick as a percentage of those economically active, 1981
ETH	% of residents born in countries of the New Commonwealth or Pakistan, 1981
PSIKREA	% of economically active population permanently sick, 1981
HHNOR	% of households without access to a car, 1981
NOAMS	% of households with no amenities, 1981
OVCD	% of households overcrowded, 1981
CN	% of households with head in social class N,1981 (N=1,...,6)
GP065	Proportion of GPs aged over 65, 1985

Source: Butts, Hancock and Swales (1989)

Measures of social deprivation were all derived from the 1981 census. The housing variables included some which reflect household composition (eg, SPAR and ELDAL) as well as those reflecting housing conditions (NOAMS and OVCD). Some of the others (eg, ETH, HHNOR etc) will be highly collinear with housing conditions. It is recognized that these data are not ideal: census data at small area level is often quickly outdated, and contains no data on homelessness, as mentioned earlier.

Information on actual death rates for electoral wards was obtained from the OPCS, and expected death rates were supplied by the

Table 3.2.   *Parameter estimates for bed-days models*

Variable	S E Thames	Wessex	Trent
	(t-statistics in parentheses)		
CONSTANT	0.19	4.09	4.10
	(0.43)	(2.31)	(6.79)
BDAYS	0.80	0.81	- - -
	(14.5)	(11.61)	
LSMR75	0.30	0.38	0.58
	(4.04)	(2.09)	(4.14)
LACCESS	0.04	0.11	0.07
	(2.22)	(5.86)	(3.67)
C1	- - -	−0.05	- - -
		(-3.01)	
C2	−0.06	−0.04	- - -
	(-3.38)	(−2.65)	
C3	- - -	−0.04	- - -
		(−2.43)	
C4	- - -	−0.04	- - -
		(−2.26)	
C5	−0.01	- - -	- - -
	(−3.48)		
ETH	0.02	- - -	- - -
	(4.14)		
HNOCAR	0.002	- - -	0.007
	(2.33)		(4.00)
MOVED	- - -	−0.01	- - -
		(−2.72)	
PSIKEA	- - -	−0.02	0.03
		(−3.42)	(2.53)
UNSK	- - -	−0.06	- - -
		(−2.91)	
GP065	- - -	- - -	0.01
			(3.14)
SPAR	- - -	- - -	-0.13
			(-3.96)
UNEMP	- - -	- - -	0.03
			(3.34)
NOAMS	- - -	- - -	0.03
			(4.14)
OVCD	- - -	- - -	-0.04
			(-4.34)
Adjusted R^2	0.43	0.40	0.48
No. of electoral wards	484	316	120

Source: Butts, Hancock and Swales (1989)
Note: Variables prefixed by 'L' are in $\log_{10}$ form

DHSS. To calculate the access scores, information on the grid references of all non-psychiatric, non-maternity NHS hospitals in each of the six RHAs was obtained manually from maps. Grid references of the geographic centroids of electoral wards were obtained from the Census. The straight line distance to each hospital from the geographical centroid of each electoral ward was calculated. Finally, information on variables proxying both the quantity and quality of GP provision was obtained from a survey of Family Practitioner Committees (Jarman 1983). Quantity of GP provision was measured by determining the average list sizes of GPs. The quality of GP provision was proxied by examining the proportions of GPs aged over 65. The presumption is that the greater this proportion, the poorer the quality of GP provision in that area. This assumption obviously requires further testing, and alternatives might include changes in SMR or consumer surveys. Data on GP provision were for 1985.

Results

Table 3.2 presents the results of estimating equation 9 for the three regions with the most reliable data. The equation was estimated using Ordinary Least Squares regression analysis. A variety of other models, including admissions and length of stay models, and models with alternative specifications have also been tested (see Butts, Hancock and Swales 1989). In addition, a wide variety of tests of specification were carried out on the model presented here (see Hancock, Holden and Swales 1990). The results reported here are those arrived at after carrying out these tests and are therefore considered the most reliable. The set of independent variables which proved to be statistically significant, for example, were arrived at using backwards elimination from a larger original set.

A number of important features are evident from these results. First, in all three regions the coefficient on the SMR variable is significantly less than 1.00. This is important because the RAWP formula imposes a value of 1.00 on the SMR variable. The implication of this finding is that resource allocation within regions is significantly less responsive to the SMR variable than resource allocation between regions. It was also found that when equality of the coefficient on SMR75 as between the three regions was tested for, the hypothesis that the coefficient was the same in all three regions could not be rejected. The value of the SMR coefficient on the pooled dataset was 0.38 (Hancock, Holden and Swales 1990).

Second, the hypothesis that a group of social variables influences the intraregional pattern of resource use in the three regions cannot be rejected. The variables which are significant and the magnitude of the coefficients on them vary considerably between the regions. However, there seems to be a very strong case for arguing that patients' home conditions, among other factors, influence the geographical pattern of the consumption of hospital resources. The RAWP formula did not include any social factors, although there was an expectation that the RHAs might wish to take such factors into account when allocating resources to DHAs (DHSS 1986, p 2). In particular, it is apparent that housing conditions have a small, but statistically significant influence in Trent region. Although arguments have been advanced in this paper why housing conditions may be a determinant of the pattern of hospital resource use, other explanations for these findings are possible. It may be for example, that the vector of social factors which has turned out to be significant is in fact a proxy for some latent, but unmeasured, variable—possibly an index of relative morbidity, and that the social variables bear a different relationship to the latent variable in each of the three regions.

Policy implications

The results of the regression models reported here simply reflect the revealed preferences and priorities of the various 'economic agents' who make up the local supply regime. They demonstrate that the local level assessment of needs for hospital resources differs from the national level view as embodied by the RAWP formula. In particular, there does seem to be a *de facto* link between patients' social conditions, including housing conditions, and the pattern of consumption of hospital resources.

In order to argue that these results have implications for the spatial allocation of command over hospital resources, at least two assumptions must be made. The first is that those who are engaged in the allocation of resources at local level are better able to evaluate relative need for such services (and act on this evaluation) than high level administrators in the DoH. The second assumption is that there is consistency amongst the results from different regions.

To accept the first assumption carries the implicit belief that those at local level have a more detailed knowledge of the conditions of patients and the potential trade-offs in their treatment than those at national level. Although this assumption seems reasonable, it could be challenged on the basis that the use of resources at the local level depends on the differential power of the individual economic agents and it is not necessarily the case that those with the most power will be aware of (and act in) the patient's best interests. If this first assumption is rejected, the analysis is still interesting but the pattern of resource use at the local level should not be used as a basis for a national resource allocation formula.

If the first assumption is accepted, however, then the second becomes important. It would be difficult to argue that the allocation of resources between regions should be determined by the priorities revealed at local level, if these priorities differed in the various regions because there would then be mutually inconsistent rules for dividing the national NHS 'cake'. In this respect, the finding that the coefficient on the deaths variable does not differ significantly across regions is important. However, it is rather more difficult to devise a national level resource allocation formula which takes account of the diverse ways in which social factors are important in the different regions.

In fact, the DHSS commissioned research for the 1986 *Review of the RAWP Formula,* using the data and general approach described in this paper (Coopers and Lybrand 1988). In commissioning this type of small area analysis, the Government have implicitly accepted that information about resource use at the local level could be used to improve the national formula for inter-regional resource allocation. Adjustments to the RAWP formula have been announced in the recent White Paper *Working for Patients* (HMSO 1989), which have explicitly incorporated earlier results from this research. The proposed changes in the white paper appear to accept the general approach that resource use can be employed to guide national level resource allocation. In particular, the white paper recommends the use of SMR to age 75 as the appropriate deaths measure, with an elasticity of 0.5,[6] and the incorporation of a weighting for social factors. In other words, resource allocation between the fourteen RHAs will be less responsive to the deaths measure, but will now change in accordance with changes in social and housing conditions. The white paper however, recommends the use of a preexisting composite indicator of social deprivation, the UPA8 index. The RAWP review argued that the absence of a specific, purpose built index of social deprivation obliged them to use indices developed for other purposes (DHSS 1988: para. 2.21). The UPA8 index is a weighted sum of eight census variables, where the weights were derived from a survey of GPs on the importance of various factors in increasing demands for their services (Jarman 1983). The variables and their weights are given in Table 3.3.

There are two problems with using this composite index. First, the variables are different from the variables which were found to be significant in the models presented here: the use of individual social variables proved to be statistically superior to the composite

Table 3.3.   Components of the UPA8 index

Variable	Weight*
ELDAL	6.19
U5	4.64
UNSK	3.74
OVCD	2.88
MOVED	2.68
ETH	2.50
SPAR	3.01
UNEMP	3.34

Source: Jarman (1983)

Note: * Each variable has previously had an arcsin
transformation applied to it to correct for 'skewness'

UPA8 index (Hancock, Holden and Swales 1990). Second, the use of a single indicator for all regions implies that each supply regime ie, region, views the need for hospital services with respect to social variables in the same way. The results presented here suggest that this is not the case.

Notwithstanding the technical criticisms that can be raised concerning the precise changes which the white paper and the RAWP review have recommended for the RAWP formula, it is clear that their effect will be explicitly to make the allocation of NHS hospital resources more responsive to geographical variations in housing and social conditions. Thus it may be argued that the *de facto* connection between health and housing is about to become, providing the general principles embodied in the white paper's recommendations for the funding of the NHS hospital service re enacted, a *de jure* one.

Notes

1   The acronym RAWP stands for Resource Allocation Working Party. Scotland and Wales have resource allocation formulae which operate on very similar principles.

2   SMR for medical condition m and sex k (SMR_{mk}) is calculated:

$$SMR_{mk} = \frac{\text{actual deaths}_{mk} \cdot 100}{\text{expected deaths}_{mk}}$$

Expected deaths$_{mk}$ is the number of regional deaths from medical condition m that would be expected for sex k ...'if the national mortality ratios by age and sex were applicable to the population of that Region' (DHSS 1976: 16). In other words, the expected figure standardizes for the region's particular age structure. An SMR_{mk} greater than 100 implies that the region's mortality rate for condition m and sex k is greater than would be expected, given the region's age structure.

3   One reason why they were not taken into account was because they were known to be collinear with deaths (DHSS 1976).

4   Postcode information was used to allocate patients' home addresses to electoral wards. There appeared to be some problems with Mersey's data, in that there were significant numbers of patient records without area of residence codes. Similarly, W Midlands appeared to have a coding problem in that 22 per cent of electoral wards had no hospital admissions. Finally, N W Thames region presents a different kind of problem in that it has very high cross-regional boundary flows. Even though it was possible to exclude electoral wards with high patient outflows, there still remains the problem that much of N W thames' hospital capacity is filled by patients resident outwith the region. Access measures are therefore unreliable for this region.

5   The result of these exclusions is to reduce the number of usable electoral wards from 3,737 to 920 (see Table 3.2). The exclusion of wards with high patient outflows and in teaching districts is wholly consistent with the purposes of the study since both these elements are funded separately in the RAWP formula.

6   It has been argued elsewhere (Butts, Hancock and Swales 1989) that the empirical and econometric justification for selecting a weight of 0.5 is extremely weak: 0.4 would be closer to the mark.

References

Butts M S, Hancock, K E, Swales, J K 1989 The measurement of needs and the spatial allocation of NHS hospital resources. *Centre for Urban and Regional Research Discussion Papers* **38** University of Glasgow, Glasgow

Coopers and Lybrand 1988 *Integrated analysis for the review of RAWP: Report to the DHSS, Sept 1988.* Coopers and Lybrand Associates, London

Department of Health and Social Security 1976 *Sharing resources for health in England. The report of the Resource Allocation Working Party (RAWP).* HMSO, London

Department of Health and Social Security 1986 *Review of the RAWP formula. Report by the NHS Management Board.* DHSS, London

Hancock K E, Holden D R, Swales J K 1990 *The consistency of the spatial allocation of NHS hospital resources: an econometric analysis.* Mimeo, University of Strathclyde, Glasgow

HMSO 1989 *Working for Patients.* Cm 555, HMSO, London

Jarman B 1983 Identification of underprivileged areas. *British Medical Journal* **286**:725–59

Mays N 1987 Measuring need in the National Health Service resource allocation formula: Standardized mortality ratios or social deprivation? *Public Administration* **65**:45–60

Smith S J 1989 Housing and health: a review and research agenda *Centre for Housing Research Discussion Papers* **27** University of Glasgow, Glasgow

PART II
HOUSING
PROVISION
FOR
'MEDICAL' NEEDS

4 Housing opportunities for people with health needs: an overview

Susan J. Smith

Housing policy and housing paths

Adequate affordable housing is generally thought of as a basic human necessity and a fundamental right of citizenship. For many people, housing is much more than bricks and mortar, and brings with it the guarantees of security, welfare and wellbeing that are themselves a condition of full participation in society. Housing however is neither uniformly serviceable nor uniformly available. The housing stock varies systematically in its character, cost, and quality over space; it varies in availability and affordability over time.

Housing policy is what mediates between an uneven stock of dwellings and those seeking a home: housing policy determines the number, type, quality and affordability of dwellings at particular times and places; it determines the balance of public and private involvement in the production, management and maintenance of the housing stock; and it determines the criteria—such as 'need' at one end of the spectrum and 'ability to pay' at the other—on which housing becomes available to populations.

In Britain housing policy serves a number of aims (see Clapham et al 1990 for more detailed discussion). It has been allied with urban policy as an instrument of environmental improvement and upgrading; it has been wielded as a form of economic management; and it has served as an aspect of social and health care policy. This chapter is concerned with the last of these facets of housing policy, and assesses the extent to which, through the social aims of housing policy (which may be realized through the market as well as state sectors of the housing system), the housing needs of people with health problems are accommodated. The aim of this chapter is to provide some context and an introduction to the second section of the book as a whole. The arguments are based on two earlier literature reviews (Smith 1989; Smith 1990). The aim here is to illustrate that there are real choices to be made between housing policies that help reproduce health inequalities and those that actively promote public health and wellbeing.

Figure 4.1 simplifies some of the complex relationships between housing and health, and shows in diagrammatic form the various routes through the different sectors of the housing market which might be followed by people with health problems. The dotted lines linking the various components of Figure 4.1 indicate the options open to households occupying different positions in housing system at the time of the onset or progression of disease, or when they are discharged from institutions or residential care but have continuing health needs.

The relationships mapped onto this diagram assume that health status interacts with housing opportunities in two key ways: via incomes; and because of the fact that some people need certain types of (supported or adapted) accommodation in order to maintain independent living. The first theme is important because there is a strong link between health, income and employment opportunities. Sick people are disproportionately poor, and poor people are disadvantaged when competing for the kind of housing to which access depends primarily on ability to pay. People with health needs are likely, then, to face problems in the market sector of the housing system, simply because of their higher than average likelihood of being unable to meet housing costs. The second theme is important because people with health problems often need to move from, or adapt, their home, in order to occupy what, for them, is a viable living space; either they need to avoid the risk factors they encounter in some housing environments (mould, damp and cold, stairs etc) or they require forms of accommodation that are not routinely supplied by the mainstream housing services (which typically cater to the average, fit, white British nuclear family).

Health problems and the housing market

The thrust of British housing policy in the last decade has been towards a market model of provision, centred around the ideology of a 'property owning democracy'. This trend is examined by Saunders (1990): it has been so successful that by the mid 1980s,

Figure 4.1. Housing paths for people with health problems

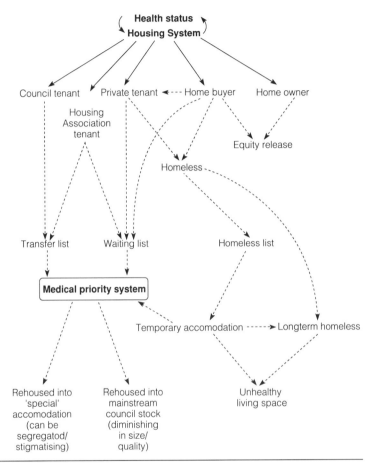

Note: The three housing queues, (transfer, waiting and homeless lists) represent routes into the social rented sector for people with health problems.

most households—around two-thirds—could be classed as owner-occupiers. This segment of the housing market is, moreover, often a profitable place in which to reside, since it is heavily 'subsidised'. Owner-occupiers receive tax relief on mortgage interest and exemption from capital gains tax for their main residence. While many people benefit from this system of housing finance, it is important to recognise that this kind of subsidy is regressive rather than progressive: the higher and more secure people's incomes, the larger their mortgage capacity (giving them an opportunity to gain maximum benefit from mortgage interest relief); and the more rapidly their dwelling appreciates, the more they benefit in financial terms from their tax exemptions from capital gain. The organization of the market sector of the housing system is not, therefore, redistributive. Neither is it aligned to the welfare ideal. The housing market deals in commercial rather than social contracts and the bottom line is ability to pay.

The housing options for home owners and buyers with health needs are indicated towards the right hand side of Figure 4.1. As long as households have had the ability to pay for home owner-ship for a good proportion of their life cycle, it is clear that home ownership can act as a significant resource for people with health needs (Leather and Wheeler 1988). For many people, poor health is associated with ageing, and illness may only begin to depress earnings capacity late in life—a time when mortgages are almost paid off, and when early retirement with relatively good benefits and guarantees is often available. For this group of sick people, early participation in the housing market represents a good invest-ment: their home, when paid for, becomes a cheap source of housing services throughout old age, and it represents a store of equity which could, if necessary, be extracted to pay for a range of social services and medical care. This role for home ownership could, with sufficient government encouragement, be set to fund a boom in the private personal social services in Britain.

Despite the advantages home ownership holds for some people with health problems, many are, nevertheless, likely to be thwart-ed in their attempts to participate—or to retain a marginal place—in the housing market. Where access to housing is controlled solely by ability to pay, we might expect people with health problems to face three kinds of difficulties.

First, it is possible that their disposable incomes will be eaten into by expenditures associated with poor health. Even with 'free' health care and exemptions from prescription costs, basic expen-ditures associated with getting about, using the home, washing, cleaning, purchasing special garments and facilities and so on, will affect the proportion of income available to meet regular housing outlays. For an owner-buyer early in a housing career, facing high interest rates, this increase in non-housing expenditure may be sufficient to prompt a move either downmarket or into the rented sector; for households outside the market sector, an illness which effectively increases the cost of living could—where these expenditures are not offset by social security payments (a problem forecast by Baldwin et al 1988)—act as a barrier to any form of owner occupation.

Second, poor health is likely to affect earning power and incomes. While chronic ill-health might exclude some people from any kind of paid employment, even intermittent ill health can restrict access to higher paying jobs, and discriminatory recruitment procedures may well exclude people with health problems from a secure place in the labour market. A characteristic of the British labour market today is its polarization into two kinds of employment. There is, on the one hand, a relatively small core of professional, managerial and commercial service workers who have secure employment and excellent fringe benefits (often including private health care). On the other hand, there is a relatively large and growing 'casualized' periphery who not only have low and unreliable income but who are also expected to take responsibility for their own insurance and sick pay arrangements. There are reasons—if we think about the relationship between health, occupational status and unemployment—to think that people with health problems will be found in disproportionate numbers in this casualized periphery of the labour market, or among the unemployed (R. Smith 1987; Smith 1990).

At a time when access to mortgage finance for owner-occupation often requires two substantial incomes, and when the continuing affordability of a home (in a period of high and often rising interest rates) requires these incomes to be dependable and regular, people with health problems are unlikely to find owner-occupation a widely available option. The problem of affordability is compounded by the fact that owner-occupation is not just about owning property; it is also, and crucially, about the maintenance of that property. This is another expenditure from limited household budgets, and one that is an absolute necessity if the home itself is to remain 'healthy'—ie warm, well ventilated and free of damp, cold, mould and other risks. It is an expenditure (which people with health problems may not be able to avoid by undertaking the work themselves) which—given changes to the grant structure for repairs, maintenance and improvements to homes (Leather and Mackintosh 1989), and not discounting the advent of initiatives like *Care and Repair* (see Harrison and Means 1990) and other home improvement agencies (Leather et al 1985; Leather and Mackintosh 1990) and provisions for home adaptations for people with physical disabilities (Statham et al

1988)—is likely to reduce the appeal of home ownership to some people with health problems.

Third, the housing market is not generally oriented towards welfare needs. It does not tend to supply homes with the range of aids, adaptations, support services and other facilities that people with health needs might require. Private contractors have, for instance, been reluctant to build speculatively for a market of people with walking, stretching and reaching difficulties (Borsay 1986). The only area of special provision that has proved attractive to market developers is the provision of sheltered housing for older people. But most schemes limit the degree of frailty, disability and other health needs they will accommodate (often requiring people to leave in very old age), and private provision for other kinds of health need is relatively rare. There are, further, concerns about the adequacies of the social security system as as a means of enabling people with health problems to maintain their private dwellings in a form suited to their medical needs (Baldwin et al 1988). Even if affordability does not become a problem, therefore, it is possible that poor health will force people to move out of owner-occupation in search of housing more suited to their condition and lifestyle.

There are likely to be problems for sick people on low incomes who seek to participate in that part of the housing system—the housing market—which has become the British cultural norm. Those who have paid off enough of their mortgage to use their home as an asset can benefit from this norm (and from the policy decisions that made it the norm), if they are prepared to release equity or trade down to realize capital (which in both cases also reduces the amount that can be transferred to families through inheritance). Others are not so fortunate: if they fail to attain, or are forced to relinquish, a home of their own, they must turn to other parts of the housing system for accommodation.

One of the Government's favoured alternatives is the small, but apparently expanding, privately rented sector. This sector, which seemed set to wither away altogether for much of the postwar period, is to be revived by the provisions of the *1988 Housing Act*. Although private renting is labelled by the new legislation as part of the 'independent' sector, it is clearly to work according to market principles. Those paying the fair market rents will still need regular and reasonable incomes if they are to sustain a decent home. Yet, if anything, the 1988 legislation made this sector more precarious for people with health problems, reducing security of tenure and making eviction much easier, especially for misdemeanours which include relatively short-term non payments of rent (Clapham et al 1990).

Housing association renting is a popular alternative to the private market, but the total housing stock managed by housing associations is small (around 600,000 dwellings, compared with the 4.5 million homes still owned by local authorities), and most of the options for people with medical needs are contained within the even smaller special needs sector (housing associations let 34,000 places in small hostels, group homes and other forms of shared housing). There is, moreover, the danger noted by Best (1988) that housing associations will trade their social role for a role as a stepping stone from the public to the private sector under the new housing legislation—even though funding changes should not affect the growth of the special needs sector.

Public sector alternatives

Given the problems of sustaining costs in the private sector, and given the size of the housing association stock, the safest option for people with health problems who cannot, or do not wish to, enter owner occupation is council renting. Housing or rehousing in the council sector is assigned on the basis of various measures of 'need', and for people with health problems, the element of need likely to carry most weight is that assigned on medical grounds. Medical priority is a long established principle of housing management in Britain. People with medical needs usually have high priority in housing queues: only homeless people and people who need to be moved to enable the existing council stock to be upgraded or cleared, tend to be housed with comparable urgency. However, some local authorities may routinely exclude some groups from applying for medical priority.

Current owner-occupiers, for instance, are often precluded from queueing for a council home at all, the tacit assumption being that they are already adequately housed. Sometimes, but not always, this exclusion is waived for people with medical needs. Likewise home owners who sell up and become homeless rather than risk repossession and eviction may be regarded by local authorities as having waived their statutory entitlement to rehousing, on the grounds that they made themselves homeless 'intentionally'. When people become homeless 'intentionally', they disqualify themselves from the housing queue, however pressing their other housing (including medical) needs.

Owner-occupiers are not the only group who may make themselves homeless in a manner which, for the purposes of the housing system, may be deemed 'intentional': women leaving violent relationships, migrants leaving their homes overseas, and people leaving their parental home may all fall into this category. The distinction between intentional and unintentional homelessness is problematic because not only are unintentionally homeless people

67

the only group who have a statutory right to housing, they are also the only group whose priority needs are defined by legislation. Homeless people should receive housing priority when they are pregnant, have dependant children, have lost their home due to an emergency such as fire or flood, or are vulnerable due to old age, mental illness or handicap, physical disability or other special reason (which, as Watchman and Robson (1990) show, case law has determined can include illness). Homeless people with health problems should therefore have few problems in gaining access not only to temporary accommodation but also to permanent rehousing, unless they made themselves homeless 'intentionally' or unless they lack a 'local connection'. This latter clause has, like the intentionally clause, been used against the interests of people with medical needs, since some local authorities still exclude people discharged, even after a long stay, from local mental institutions, from access to the local housing stock, on the grounds that their 'permanent' residence is in another district.

In theory, then, the bottom right hand corner of Figure 4.1 should be empty: no sick people should be found among the long term homeless, and anyone with health needs in temporary accommodation should very quickly move on. In practice, as the diagram indicates, there are a number of ways in which sick people may end up either spending long periods in temporary accommodation, or simply living on the street (these are outlined in more detail in Shanks and Smith, in press). As a consequence the health profile of homeless people is increasingly distinctive, and the poor health of people who fail to find a permanent home is exacerbated by harsh living environments as well as by their limited access to primary medical care (an issue taken up in Part III of this volume).

Notwithstanding some inequalities and, probably, injustices, in who may queue for a council home, once people are deemed eligible, there is a well developed system in Britain of assigning housing priority in the public sector on health grounds. This is usually referred to as the medical priority system (though it is anything but *a* system, and practices vary widely from local authority to local authority). The role and relevance of building medical priority into housing allocations systems is considered by Connelly and Roderick in Chapter 5, and is currently being reviewed on a national scale (Smith, McGuckin and Walker 1991). It is therefore only necessary to make two key points here concerning the housing opportunities this system holds for people with health problems or medical needs.

First, it is important to note that the outcome of medical priority assignations may differ according to whether the applicant is homeless, queueing on the general waiting list, or applying for a transfer within the council rented stock. Because of the marked increase in homelessness in Britain over the last fifteen years, and in the light of the statutory obligations local authorities have to rehouse this group, homeless queues are usually the longest, and move fastest, in the rehousing process. Homeless people with health problems may therefore get rehoused more quickly if they queue simply as homeless, effectively bypassing (or being excluded from) medical priority queues. But this does not necessarily mean that they will get a suitable home. Homeless people are frequently required to accept the first offer issued to them, or lose their place in the housing queue. Housing managers, whose goal is to let as much of the stock as possible as quickly as possible, will therefore tend to offer homeless people accommodation in the areas and properties which are in least demand from other applicants—often in 'difficult to let' estates—a label that is usually synonymous with 'unhealthy housing'. This could mean that a history of homelessness will continue to drive health inequalities, even when once-homeless people move back into the mainstream housing stock.

Additionally, people with medical needs who are already council tenants and require a transfer are often considered separately from people queueing with medical priority on the waiting lists. Sometimes, existing tenants are excluded from the same kind of medical priority as waiting list applications (the assumption being that the very fact of residence in council housing exempts them from certain kinds of health problem, eg those stemming from the condition of the home). The implications of this for the relative chances of the two groups of getting a move to an appropriate dwelling has yet to be established, but it may be important.

Second, the medical priority system is still something of a 'black box'. Given the extent to which it dominates local authority housing decisions it is surprising how little investigation there has so far been of how fairly and effectively allocations procedures discriminate between people who are 'sick' and those who are 'well' (especially if we consider how much attention has been given to whether and how that system discriminates between people who are 'black' and 'white' and between men and women). There is no common practice concerning how much weight to assign medical priority relative to other priority claims, and there are wide variations in just how people with medical priority queue: some queue in separate categories; some gain points which are weighed alongside every one else's points; some wait in an order dictated by one or more priority labels; some simply queue in date order. Just how these different systems sort medical priority applicants and match them to available property still has to be established. Whether some groups are advantaged relative, to others, and whether this advantage is 'just' or 'rational' is also open to question. What we do know is that there are essentially two routes out of the medical priority system, and that these reflect differences in health status as well as dwelling supply.

A minority of medical priority applicants are rehoused into 'special' schemes which may be managed either by the local authority or by local housing associations. The pros and cons of 'special' housing are reviewed elsewhere (Borsay 1988; Cook 1984; Clapham and Smith 1990). This sector is dominated by provision for older people, and to a lesser extent specializes in homes for people with mental health problems and learning difficulties. Demand even from these carefully circumscribed groups exceeds special housing supply in many areas (Lipscombe 1987), and there seems little scope for extending the special needs label to homes for the wide variety of vulnerable groups considered by Cook (1984). The 'special' route out of the medical priority system is therefore rather restricted, though it does bring the promise of relatively new homes, with relatively good facilities and a relatively wide range of services. This increasingly contrasts with the second route: rehousing into the mainstream council rented stock.

The majority of medical priority applicants are rehoused, if at all, and sometimes after a long wait, into the existing general needs council housing stock. There are a number of difficulties here, in addition to waiting time which can itself be a health risk for some people. Waiting time may be long where the applicant requests, or is advised by doctors to take, a particular kind of dwelling such as ground floor accommodation and in a particular kind of area (eg near to a special school). Other problems arise because the medical priority applicant must queue alongside people with many other priority claims for a home in a stock which is diminishing in size and quality. Many local authorities thus find their lists dominated by applications from homeless people. Also they may be subject to a variety of political pressures, for instance to supply homes for 'sons and daughters' of existing tenants. At a time when housing supply was abundant, these competing claims might not compromise a commitment to medical priority: as supply diminishes, however, the prioritizing of different kinds of needs may not necessarily work to the advantage of people with health problems.

Conclusion

This chapter has offered an overview of the different housing circumstances and options that people with medical needs might encounter on their life path. British housing policy is not—and does not aspire to be—tenure neutral. The aim is to promote the market generally, and owner-occupation in particular. Indeed,the aim is even more specific—to promote a particular form of owner occupation based on the individualized consumption of private property. The wealth transfers (through taxation and subsidy) that underpin this system are not progressive, and while this approach to housing finance guarantees that ownership is the preferred, and, indeed, economically most beneficial option for most citizens, it is clear that people with health problems can lose out, either because they cannot compete in the market place, or because the market does not provide, at an affordable price, the housing 'goods' they require. This is unfortunate, but it is neither unpredictable nor inevitable. There is no economic reason (though there are political and ideological reasons) why home ownership cannot be subsidised progressively; there is no reason why shared or group, rather than individual, home ownership (or housing cooperatives) could not be developed to allow the costs as well as the benefits of ownership to be shared, and there is no reason why there could not be more public investment into the public rented sector to ensure that it remains a safety net for those who must—as well as those who choose to—rent. The important fact to bear in mind when reading the chapters which follow, then, is that the housing opportunities available to people with medical needs are a product of political choices. Choices that can be challenged, and could be changed.

References

Baldwin S, Parker G, Walker R Eds 1988 *Social security and community care.* Avebury, Aldershot

Best R 1988 Community care and housing associations. In Baldwin S, Parker G, Walker R Eds 1988 *Social security and community care.* Avebury, Aldershot, 37–42

Borsay A 1988 *Disabled people in the community. A study of housing, health and welfare services.* Bedford Square Press, London

Cook F 1984 Housing special groups. *Housing Review* **33**: 208–12

Clapham D, Kemp P, Smith S J 1990 *Housing and social policy.* Macmillan, Basingstoke and London

Clapham D, Smith S J 1990 Housing policy and 'special needs'. *Policy and Politics* **18**: 193–206

Harrison L, Means R 1990 *Housing. The essential element in community care.* Anchor Housing Trust, Oxford

Leather P, Mackintosh S 1989 The means testing of improvement grants. *Housing Review* **38**: 77–80

Leather P, Mackintosh S 1990 *Monitoring assisted agency services: Part 1, home improvement agencies—an evaluation of performance*, HMSO, London

Leather P, Murie A, Hayes L, Bishop J 1985 *Review of home improvement agencies.* Department of the Environment, London

Leather P, Wheeler R 1988 *Making use of home equity in old age.* Building Societies Association, London

Lipscomb D 1987 *Losing patients: a report on priority groups.* Greater London Association of Community Health Councils, London

Saunders P 1990 *A nation of home owners.* Unwin Hyman, London

Shanks N, Smith S J in press. Public policy and the health of homeless people. *Policy and Politics* forthcoming

Smith R 1987 *Unemployment and health.* Oxford University Press, Oxford

Smith S J 1989 Housing and health: a review and research agenda. *Discussion Paper* 27. Centre for Housing Research, Glasgow University

Smith S J 1990 Health status and the housing system. *Social Science and Medicine* **31**: 753–62

Smith S J, McGuckin A, Walker C 1991 Housing provision people with health problems. Paper presented to the conference: *Unhealthy housing: the public health response.* University of Warwick

Statham R, Korczak J, Monaghan P 1988 *House adaptations for people with physical disabilities.* HMSO, London

Watchman P O, Robson P 1989 *Homelessness and the law in Britain.* Planning Exchange, Glasgow

5 Medical priority for rehousing: an audit

Jim Connelly and
Paul Roderick

Although housing policy has been central to public health reform since the mid-nineteenth century, the present day medical profession has only a vestigial interest, which is largely confined to the system of 'medical priority for rehousing' (MPR). This is despite the growing housing crisis in the UK, and calls for a greater involvement by the medical profession in recognising the impact of housing on health inequalities (Morris 1990).

In principle MPR is a mechanism whereby 'medical need' is taken account of in the welfare provision of public sector housing. Although there is variation in the procedures adopted by local authorities, MPR is most commonly achieved by the assignment of points, which contribute to the priority for rehousing. The current involvement of the medical profession in housing decisions takes two forms: advice to housing departments and/or assessment of applicants by public health physicians, and the provision of supporting information about specific applicants by general practitioners or hospital consultants. The role of public health physicians stems from the joint arrangements (between local authorities and health authorities) set up in 1974 following the demise of the post of the Medical Officer of Health (MOH).

Mounting pressure on public sector housing exists because the supply has dwindled, not only for those with ill health (this includes those with 'special needs', for example people with learning difficulties), but also for homeless people and for those with social reasons for requesting rehousing or transfer. In the light of this housing shortage the MPR system itself has been criticized as being ineffective, inefficient and inequitable, and public health physicians have expressed doubts about the appropriateness of their role (Muir Gray 1978; Parsons 1987; Faculty of Public Health Medicine 1990a). Moreover, the practice of medicine has entered a more critical phase, with both intraprofessional and external evaluation of its effectiveness. Medical audit, the regular evaluation of medical care against standard criteria, has now been formalized in the current NHS reforms as a requirement of all doctors and NHS hospitals.

This paper is written against this background of the restructuring of housing and health services, and it attempts to answer the following questions:

1   What is the relationship between housing and health for the purpose of allocating medical priority?
2   What are the pressures on the rationing of public sector accommodation?
3   What evidence exists about the value of the MPR system?
4   What are the implications for the medical profession in its efforts to support improved housing conditions both for specific individuals and for the population as a whole?

Our work is informed both by a literature review and by the results of a survey of public health physicians (PHPs) undertaken in 1989 for the Housing and Health Working Party of the Faculty of Public Health Medicine (Faculty of Public Health Medicine 1990a, Roderick et al 1990).

Relationship between housing and health in the context of medical priority for rehousing (MPR)

There are two implicit assumptions underlying the medical priority system: first, that an individual's housing need is partly determined by the interaction between their current housing conditions and their state of health; and second, that it is possible to weight this need both between different individuals and against other determinants of housing need. Are such assumptions justified?

Few would dispute the considerable historical evidence which links poor housing conditions of nineteenth century urban areas with high infant and childhood mortality, and with recurrent infectious disease epidemics. More recent epidemiological studies have demonstrated associations between specific housing conditions, such as dampness and overcrowding, and various aspects of physical and mental health. These are reviewed in Muir Gray (1979) and Lowry (1990a).

Such findings vary in their robustness, partly because of the difficulties of separating the independent contribution of housing from the effects of environmental and socioeconomic factors on health: a problem which is particularly true for nonpsychotic mental illness (for example anxiety and mild depression), though some dispute the relationship altogether (Hodgson 1975). But there is, on balance, a body of evidence linking poor housing conditions and ill health. The World Health Organization (WHO) has formally acknowledged the essential contribution that decent secure accommodation makes to promoting health. Using the holistic view of health which encompasses physical, mental and social wellbeing, the WHO state:

> Over and above their basic purpose of providing shelter against the elements and a focus for family life, human dwellings should afford protection against the hazard to health arising from the physical and social environments. At its best housing promotes physical and mental health. It provides people with psychological security, physical ties with their community and culture and a means of expressing their individuality. (World Health Organization 1989).

The 'Health Field Concept of Health', which has been influential in formulating health promotion policy, describes four influences on health : genetic predisposition, environment, lifestyle, and the health care system. This perspective likewise explicitly recognizes housing as a central determinant of health (Lalonde 1984). However, a central theoretical difficulty remains both in extrapolating results from epidemiological studies to individuals, and in attempting to impute a casual relationship between housing and health. For example, while several studies have demonstrated a link between dampness and self-reported wheezing, this does not mean that an individual living in a damp house who complains of wheezing can definitely have this attributed to dampness.

While recognizing this difficulty, for the purposes of assigning medical priority, the logical relationships between housing and health have been categorized. Muir Gray (1979) describes five categories:

1 Housing directly influencing physical health;
2 Housing directly influencing mental health;
3 Illness leading to housing problems;
4 Housing factors which complicate an illness;
5 A combination of the above.

Although research has concentrated on exploring the first two relationships, most applicants for medical priority lie in the third and fourth categories. Moreover there is now substantial *a priori* reason and empirical evidence linking ill health to the conditions in temporary accommodation—such as 'bed and breakfast' hotels. Temporary accommodation is widely used by local authorities carrying out their statutory duties to priority homeless households. It is ironic then that such ill health has been the consequence not the

75

cause of the prioritization of housing need. Furthermore, the detrimental influence of the environmental conditions faced by the single homeless, who are usually denied MPR support and who do not constitute a statutory 'priority group', is even more evident. Many of these individuals would fit into category five, for example, due to pre-existing mental illness.

In practice the MPR system seems to be dominated by the problems of older people suffering from acquired physical disability. For example, in Bolton, in 251 applicants rehoused through the MPR system the following groups of disorders were found: cardiovascular/neurological disorders (eg angina, stroke) in 36 per cent, musculoskeletal diseases (eg osteoarthritis) in 24 per cent, respiratory problems in 12 per cent and psychiatric disorders in 6 per cent (Cole 1986). The majority were over 65 years of age. Similarly, in Oldham, over 50 per cent of applicants had cardiovascular disease or arthritis and 60 per cent were over 65 years of age (Gardner 1981).

The major reason given for requesting rehousing is reduced mobility; for example amongst applicants in Portsmouth who stated a specific reason, 43 per cent wanted ground floor accommodation and 30 per cent said their main problem was negotiating stairs (Howells 1984). Nationally the Department of the Environment waiting list survey found that in 34 per cent of new tenants over 55 years of age, the reason for wishing to move was classified as medical handicap and 29 per cent had requested ground floor one level accommodation: comparable percentages for all ages were 11 per cent and 9 per cent respectively (Prescott-Clarke 1988).

The age distribution and pattern of medical problems found in these studies may be explained by the dramatic shift in disease patterns in the UK over the last 50 years, and by the parallel improvement in life expectancy. Infectious diseases such as diphtheria, previously causes of high infant and childhood mortality, have all but disappeared.Chronic disorders now predominate as causes of both severe morbidity and mortality in an increasingly elderly population. The recent OPCS *Survey of Disability in Adults* estimates that there are now six million people with some disability in Britain: 2.36 million are graded five or above on a ten-point severity scale; and overall 14 per cent of private households contain someone with a disability (OPCS 1988). The prevalence of disability, particularly for severe grades, rises substantially with age and is commoner in females: 69 per cent of disabled people are over 60 years of age, 56 per cent are widows whereas only 20 per cent are widowers. The most common disability is locomotor (see Table 5.1) and musculoskeletal disorders (eg osteoarthritis) are the most frequently reported causes of this disability (in 46 per

Table 5.1. *Estimates of the number of adults affected by common disabilities in private households* in Great Britain*

	000s
Locomotion	4,005
Hearing	2,365
Personal care	2,129
Dexterity	1,572
Sight	1,384
Intellect	1,183
Behaviour	1,172
Reach/stretch	1,085
Communication	989
Continence	957

Source: *OPCS surveys of disability in Great Britain* Report 1 1988.

Note: * ie excluding institutions

cent), followed by circulatory disorders (eg coronary heart disease), and respiratory disorders (eg chronic bronchitis).

There is also an increasing social class gradient in most chronic diseases, which persists in older people (Davey-Smith 1990). Moreover, those with disability have a lower chance of employment and even in work have a lower income (Office of Population Censuses and Surveys 1988). Such disparities reduce the opportunities to participate in the private housing market. In this OPCS survey 54 per cent of disabled people were not in owner occupation compared to 41 per cent of the general population. Ill health can therefore be a barrier to certain housing tenures and to improved housing conditions (Smith 1990).

Given these factors, it is inevitable that there are a large number of public sector occupants with disabilities, whose housing conditions result in substantial handicaps (ie in a limitation of their social role). Two main problems are found: the limitation of mobility if there are stairs or a hill to climb, and the inability to use household amenities (eg WC). Such disabilities may be the consequence of several underlying diseases, for example, reduced mobility from breathlessness secondary to heart failure, or chronic bronchitis, or from partial paralysis due to stroke, or from a painful hip due to osteoarthritis.

Table 5.2. *New housing starts in England and Wales*

	Public sector	Private	Total
1978	110,868	161,597	272,465
1983	53,831	179,112	232,943
1988	31,710	223,490	255,200

Source: *Housing and Construction Statistics* Department of the Environment 1989.

The complex interactions which transform disability to handicap depend not only on the underlying medical disease (and its severity and natural history) and particular housing conditions, but also fundamentally on social factors such as support—by family, friends or agencies—and income. Is it possible therefore, to separate and weight the effects of housing on health? Parsons found that there was little agreement between medical officers in allocation of medical priority (Parsons 1987). Some have concluded that weighting is not possible and simply allocate the same number of points irrespective of the underlying problem (Muir Gray 1978). Others adopt some form of scale (Howells 1984). In principle any weighting should be based on an objective assessment of the applicant's handicap and not on their 'disease' alone, together with their potential to benefit from rehousing.

Pressure on public sector accommodation

Application for MPR is common practice: in the Department of the Environment's waiting list survey, 23 per cent of waiting list applicants had stated a medical problem and 8 per cent thought the council had accepted this as a reason for priority (Prescott-Clarke 1988). However MPR is only one aspect of the management of public sector housing demand, and must therefore be seen in this overall context. Households may apply for rehousing if they are new tenants—not previously in council accommodation; or for a transfer if they are existing tenants. Reasons given include living in accommodation which lacks basic amenities (eg inside WC), or which is in poor condition (eg damp, overcrowded), or difficulty with access to services (eg shops, relatives), and homelessness. Medical problems can be taken into account in two ways: as legitimate criteria for being deemed in priority need under the homelessness legislation or through priority being ascribed within the MPR system.

Table 5.3. *Employment status of people on council waiting lists*

	On list	Not on list
Employed full-time	340 (45%)	11,920 (62%)
Employed part-time	40 (5%)	800 (4%)
Unemployed	130 (17%)	1,430 (7%)
Retired	110 (14%)	2,470 (13%)
Permanently sick disabled	40 (5%)	500 (3%)
Inactive	100 (13%)	2,210 (11%)

Source: Housing Trailers to the 1981 and 1984 Labour Force Surveys Department of the Environment 1988.

Public sector provision has changed dramatically in the last decade, primarily due to government policy. The fragile post war consensus which saw this sector as an essential element of the welfare state has been replaced by an increased emphasis on the private sector, with owner-occupation becoming the favoured form of provision. The role of local authorities in providing housing has been constrained, and consequently there has been a substantial reduction in the building of new public sector homes, not matched by the 40 per cent expansion of the private sector over the same period, see Table 5.2. Housing associations have also been squeezed, the number of new starts falling from 18,217 in 1978 to 9,690 in 1988, although they are now seen as the favoured form of low cost or subsidised rented housing.

Moreover the 1980 Housing Act (1981 in Scotland) gave tenants the opportunity to buy their home from local authorities, new towns or housing associations under favourable terms. By 1988 over 1.4 million homes were bought under such 'right to buy' schemes in England and Wales (Department of the Environment 1989a). Such dwellings are thereby removed from the public sector and, perhaps not surprisingly the properties remaining are in the least favourable location and in the poorest condition, such as inner city high rise flats. Council accommodation is now a marker of social status, and those on council waiting lists are likely to be socioeconomically deprived with a high level of unemployment and low income amongst applicants (Prescott-Clark et al 1988) see Table 5.3

Pressure for public sector accommodation has been further exacerbated by an estimated 10 per cent rise in the number of census defined households, in England and Wales, from 18.196 million in 1981 to 19.99 million by 1991 (Department of the Environment 1989a). If potential households are also taken into account the latter figure increases by 1.2 million (Niner 1989).

The growing mismatch between supply and demand for public sector housing and the inaccessibility of owner occupation for many has inevitably lead to an increase in homelessness. The number of households officially accepted annually as homeless in England has risen from 53,100 in 1978 to over 126,680 in 1989 (Department of the Environment 1989b). The 1989 figure represents nearly half a million people. Local authorities have a duty to rehouse households accepted as statutorily homeless under the terms of the *1985 Housing Act*, but there is an even greater number without access to independent decent accommodation who are not accepted for rehousing under this legislation. Such households such as childless couples constitute the 'hidden homeless', estimated in London to be three to four times greater than the 'official homeless' figure (Faculty of Public Health Medicine 1991) and to number two million nationally (Shelter 1990). The true scale of the problem facing public sector housing managers is shown by the *1984 Labour Force Survey* which provides the most accurate estimate of the waiting list (Department of the Environment 1988). Three quarters of a million households were waiting for council properties, with an additional half a million requesting transfer. The problems have undoubtedly worsened since this survey was completed.

A more recent development has been 'special needs housing' (Lowry 1990b). This is specifically targeted at groups such as those with learning difficulties, who may in general have particular needs for housing and social support, and who are thought to need positive discrimination in housing allocation. Such need has arisen from the shift in social policy to provide 'care in the community' rather than institutional care. In London such a 'special needs' policy has also been recommended for the rising problem of single homelessness which has been exacerbated by the closure of hostels (Llewelyn-Davies 1990). Housing associations are key providers in this field, receiving central funding—from the Housing Corporation, and local funding from health and local authorities. However the definition and separation of such broad groups of special need is not based on individual needs. It has been argued that it is inequitable and also criticized as stigmatizing and ineffective in delivering 'care by the community' which would increase individual autonomy (Clapham and Smith and 1990). Nevertheless such a policy does at least focus attention and specific funding on deprived groups. In principle, local authorities could use their nomination rights to secure accommodation for appropriate applicants on their waiting lists.

In summary applicants for rehousing or transfer with medical problems are facing competing pressures for a dwindling supply of public sector accommodation. Inevitably, in these circumstances, there may have been a tendency to use medical priority as a method of increasing the chances of rehousing success. In particular those not using the medical priority system, or denied access to it, may have as legitimate an argument for better housing based on the interaction of their current accommodation with their state of health.

Medical priority—how can it be evaluated?

Any assessment of the value of the MPR system must start from the aims and objectives of the system. For medical priority the implicit aim is to take account of 'medical need' in the allocation of priority for rehousing. However 'need' is not an absolute concept but a complex construction. It requires qualification as 'need for', the 'for' referring to a specific intervention. Need can also be constructed from different perspectives: applicant, housing officer, health professional, relative, politician. These may differ substantially. For example Kohli (1986), in a survey in Edinburgh, found that general practitioners awarded more priority points to individuals than did public health physicians.

From the medical perspective allocation of priority can be viewed as a 'prescription of rehousing', analogous for example to surgery or drug prescribing (Muir Gray 1979; Hodgson 1975). Such decision making is at the core of medical practice. The decision may be easy, where the diagnosis is clear cut, the management options limited, and the intervention beneficial, for example when orthopaedic surgery is required for fractured neck of femur. In other cases it may be more difficult to determine the balance of risk and benefit.

Several authors view MPR as a component of medical rehabilitation (Hodgson 1975; Cole 1986). This perspective seeks to make a diagnosis not only of any specific disease and resulting disability, but also on how the applicant's accommodation (defined by size, type, site, amenities, conditions) interacts to produce handicap. This paradigm considers how the disability might change over time—requiring an understanding of the natural history of the condition; weighs up the alternatives such as provision of home aids; and,if rehousing is thought appropriate, it prescribes a specific form of housing which overall would give greater benefit than costs for the applicant. Some practitioners have made such a prescription down to the detail of the height of sink or switches (Hodgson 1975).

To evaluate the MPR system, whatever the medical perspective adopted, we require criteria by which such an intervention can be judged. Maxwell (1984) has defined six criteria:

81

1 Equity
2 Effectiveness
3 Efficiency
4 Acceptability
5 Accessibility
6 Relevance to need

In an equally influential conceptual model, Donabedian (1966) divided medical care interventions into three components:

Structure (eg staff, resources)
Process (eg procedures, activity) and
Outcome (eg lives saved, changes in patients' quality of life)

Evaluation can be at any of these three levels and should involve comparing the actual practice with standards set within each criterion examined. Some of these concepts are now applied to the evaluation of the MPR system.

Equity

This is one of the most important criteria if housing allocation is to be on the basis of need. The priority system assumes unequal needs require unequal treatment. However there is evidence, first, of geographical inequity in both the process of medical priority and, less certainly, the outcome. Such inequity stems from the wide variation in the systems of assessment and points allocation used which may, in turn, reflect a lack of agreed standards. Thomas (1978) reported that in 39 Welsh local authorities 29 used a points system for awarding medical priority; whereas in four allocation was decided by committee; and in six there was a first come first served system. Moreover in six authorities using the points system, the maximum medical contribution to the qualifying number of points for rehousing varied from 13–67 per cent (mean 37). Such variation confirms the Department of the Environment's own research which showed that nationally there was wide discretion in the administration of council waiting lists (Prescott-Clarke 1988).

Parsons (1987) reviewed the practice of data collection in 55 local authorities: 29 per cent assessed medical priority on the basis of applicants' self-report; 22 per cent used the general practitioner; 25 per cent a health visitor home visit; and the remainder a home visit by a housing officer. Many local authorities do not have standard forms for applicants, and some specify inclusion criteria based on medical conditions rather than on resulting handicaps and even here there is inconsistency (Faculty of Public Health Medicine 1990a).

The resulting confusion may be compounded for district health authorities whose boundaries include more than one local authority because they may have to deal with different policies in each (Faculty of Public Health Medicine 1990a). Nevertheless some Directors of Public Health have worked closely with their local authorities to develop standardized procedures for application and assessment.

As well as geographical inequity there is also evidence of social inequity. The Commission for Racial Equality (CRE) found evidence of racial discrimination in the management of council lists in both Hackney and Liverpool (CRE 1984, 1988). In both places black applicants were more likely to be allocated to older properties with less amenities (eg central heating), and medical priority was less often cited for them. The findings in Hackney were thought to be representative of most urban areas, whilst in Liverpool because medical cases and decants (tenants moved because of slum clearance) were given priority for new builds, this may have exacerbated the racial inequity. Furthermore, any system that relies on applicants self-reports could introduce a selection effect which may be indirectly discriminatory, as it may favour those who are more aware of the system or those who speak English as their first language. Moreover, general practitioners may support an application *de novo* or if requested by housing officers or PHPs, and inevitably there is discretion in their responses.

In summary the large degree of discretion within the present system is likely to mean that those applying for medical priority represent the tip of an iceberg of an equally legitimate but unmet pool of people with medical needs.

Effectiveness

The effectiveness of MPR can be assessed in three ways relating to the following questions. First, does being allocated medical priority increase the chance of rehousing? This is a 'process' measure which will depend on the relative weighting in a points system or the relative importance of a medical priority category ascription in another queueing system. Second, does MPR discriminate between those with and without handicap amongst applicants for rehousing? Third, and most importantly, is there evidence that rehousing results in an overall improvement in quality of life?

Process measures

Muir Gray (1978) reviewed 612 applicants for rehousing who were referred to him in one year, in his role as community physician. Only 29 (5 per cent) were ultimately rehoused. However, this was not surprising as medical need provided only five out of a possible 30 points. He argued that the policy would be more effective if medical reasons were given greater weighting. Howells (1984) reviewed a consecutive series of 100 applicants for both rehousing and transfer three years later: 41 per cent with medical priority had been rehoused compared to 36 per cent with none (not a significant difference). This was, however, a higher rate than in Muir Gray's study as medical priority points could contribute up to 40 per cent of housing allocation points. Another study found that only 52 per cent of those given urgent medical priority had been rehoused in three years (Gardner 1981).

It appears then that being ascribed medical priority has only a limited impact on the chance of rehousing. Nor does it necessarily discriminate between severity of handicap. Maclennan et al (1982) found that a group of older people assigned medical priority were no more handicapped that the general population of the elderly, and Elton and Packer (1986) found that anxiety and depression were equally common in those requesting MPR on grounds of mental ill health and in those who did not.

Outcome measures

There is a dearth of studies addressing the question of whether rehousing improves the quality of life of applicants, particularly in comparison with those not given priority, or those not applying. Few researchers use objective measures of physical or mental health, and none have addressed the possibly disruptive effect of noninstitutional rehousing, particularly in older people. It must be recognized that such evaluation is difficult because the relationship between housing and health is complex, and consequently, the benefit of rehousing for one aspect of health may lead to a disbenefit in others, for example provision of ground floor accommodation because of mobility problems in an area which is further from relatives or where there is a higher incidence of vandalism. Moreover, the natural history of many conditions which lead to handicap is for deterioration over time, so the independent efficacy of rehousing, if it existed, will be difficult to detect.

In one study, nevertheless, the outcome of rehousing cases where the housing conditions were assessed as exacerbating the handicap of people with existing disability, was taken as self-evident (Muir Gray 1978). In another study Maclennan et al (1982) used health visitors to assess a group of older people who had been rehoused: 70 per cent of those with limited mobility and 90 per cent of those with no limitation were assessed as 'improved'. These levels were slightly higher than the subjects' self-reports, but the main reasons for self-reported dissatisfaction were social, such as being placed too far from relatives. In a similar vein a three year follow-up of people rehoused in Bolton, using self-report, found that of the 150 traced, 57 (23 per cent) reported improvement and were satisfied, 58 (23 per cent) were unchanged but satisfied, and 35 (14 per cent) unchanged and dissatisfied (Cole 1986). The commonest reason for satisfaction was the removal of the need to climb stairs, the converse was true in those who were dissatisfied.

The only study to use the formal scientific approach of a randomized controlled trial (Elton and Packer 1986, 1987) focussed on rehousing on the grounds of mental ill health. Fifty-six applicants for MPR were randomly allocated to receive MPR or not. First, of the 28 matched pairs, those given priority were more likely to be rehoused. In the 11 pairs where the priority case had been rehoused for over 12 months and the nonpriority case not rehoused, there were significant differences in anxiety and depression scores, suggesting that rehousing could improve mental ill health. However among an age–sex matched control group of housing applicants not applying for medical priority who had had similar baseline levels of anxiety and depression, it was found that rehousing improved their mental health to a similar extent. This was a small study which was not blinded, so caution is required in drawing firm conclusions. It does however illustrate the selective nature of the MPR system and the potential unmet need. This is recognised by Directors of Public Health, several of whom specifically stated in a recent survey that they doubted the effectiveness of MPR and one reported that 'nothing ever happened so I've given it up' (Roderick et al 1991)

Limitations to the effectiveness of MPR

It is important to recognise the structural constraints which may affect the effectiveness of rehousing as reported in the literature. Predominant is the lack of suitable accommodation. For example, in Glasgow over 6,000 people were assigned priority per year with only 1,000–1,250 properties becoming available, and there was a shortage of ground floor accommodation (Fisk 1982). This can mean that effective policy making is impossible and that only very urgent needs can be met (Faculty of Public Health Medicine 1990a).

A further contributing factor is the inadequacy of the medical assessment. In many there is no home visit which is compounded by the poor information received from GPs, for example in one authority nine per cent of GP/consultant support letters contained no medical information at all (Fisk 1982). Kohli (1986) surveyed GPs in Edinburgh and showed that their knowledge of the system was limited and their expectations inappropriate.

Efficiency

The notion of 'efficiency' is taken here to refer to whether the time and resources devoted to running a system maximises the output (eg applicants assessed), irrespective of the overall value of the procedure in terms of outcome. Several public health practitioners have emphasised the considerable workload for public health departments involved in assessing applications. Muir Gray (1978) spent on average half an hour per day, and Hodgson (1975) spent one day per week. This is borne out by the survey of DPHs (Roderick et al 1991). There was a high level of involvement with 73 per cent (143) departments having some input into medical priority. Of the 93 departments who reported a 'formal commitment' to housing work, the time allocated varied from one session (about four hours) per month to ten per week, with a median of one session per week. It is not known how this use of resources relates to any outcome. Only a minority reported involvement in other housing activities such as with joint care planning groups, homelessness or developing links with housing associations. Several DPHs stated that the system was a waste of their time and they were trying to reduce their input, some to concentrate on giving greater input into local housing policy (Faculty of Public Health Medicine 1990a).

The GPs role may also be inefficient. They may be asked to provide information by the applicant, housing officer, PHP, or may write in support *de novo* and there are usually no clear criteria for such housing letters. Not surprisingly the resulting information provided is often not relevant for the assessment of priority (Fisk 1982; Maclennan 1982).

Acceptability

There is little published research on the acceptability of the MPR system for applicants. The disgruntlement of many PHPs has been mentioned above, although not all decry the value of MPR, some seeing it as worthwhile for people with disability. Kohli (1986) felt that the lack of feedback to GPs was unacceptable and Fisk (1982) reported the dissatisfaction of housing officers, which stemmed primarily from the poor quality of information on which they had to base assessments.

Accessibility

The accessibility of MPR can be measured in terms of the ease by which applicants can submit applications, and the waiting time before they are given a decision and rehoused. These factors vary substantially between local authorities as has been described above. One survey found an average waiting time for council applicants of 1.8 years, but for those allocated MPR it was even higher, at two years, (Prescott-Clarke et al 1988).

Relevance to need (appropriateness)

In medical care the 'appropriateness' of a specific intervention has been studied by peer review of actual or hypothetical decision making. Consensus criteria for 'appropriateness', are ultimately derived from the medical literature concerning the treatment of the condition: Who benefits from which treatment at what cost?. There is little empirical evidence concerning the appropriateness of MPR, although studies cited above, which showed new tenant dissatisfaction (eg Cole 1986) perhaps illustrate how neglected this area is.

Any assessment of the appropriateness of MPR for an individual must consider the alternatives available and the opportunity costs of taking one option rather than another. For an individual the act of rehousing would be inappropriate if the provision of housing aids or social support in the original home could overcome the handicap more cost-effectively. Moreover, even if rehousing is required, the site, type and relevant amenities need to be specifically designated if the handicaps identified are to be ameliorated. To do otherwise would be inappropriate. For example, to rehouse someone with severe mobility problems to a first floor flat with no lift, would not, however fine the dwelling, be relevant to need. The wider issue of the appropriateness of MPR for the population raises the question of whether the time and effort spent running this system could be used more effectively to improve housing conditions overall. The DPH survey highlighted the concern of many DPHs that involvement in rationing of housing for individuals was an inappropriate task for their departments, whose role might rather be to influence local housing policy.

Conclusion

The medical priority system must be viewed in the context of the crisis in public sector housing provision in the UK. There is increasing demand from several sources, all of which have legitimate social and/or medical reasons for needing better housing. It is therefore especially important that a rehousing system at the individual level is equitable and effective. Moreover, any practitioners with involvement in MPR have a duty to evaluate their work on such criteria. Unfortunately, the overall lack of clear guidelines and objective methods of assessment in the MPR system has resulted in inequity. There may be too much local discretion, and although the evidence is scanty, the present system appears to be ineffective in obtaining rehousing for many people with medical needs. Its potential effectiveness is, in short, severely limited by the shortage of suitable accommodation. In consequence, there exists both substantial unmet need for more appropriate housing on medical grounds and evidence of the inappropriate use of the MPR system. This raises the question of whether MPR should be abolished as some suggest (Lowry 1990b) or whether it can be reformed.

In the present UK housing system there does appear to be a need for a mechanism which explicitly recognises that individuals with disabilities can be handicapped by inappropriate housing. The 'ageing' of the UK population will increase this problem, and even where 'special needs' programmes for older people exist they may fail to respond to individual housing needs.

For an individual the relationship between housing and health is likely to be complex and, therefore, a cursory assessment of needs based on self-report health is probably an insufficient basis for housing decisions. A full assessment of housing conditions in the context of physical and mental health together with social and environmental factors would be the ideal, with explicit consideration of alternatives to rehousing. Such a system would entail close cooperation and integration between housing departments and social services, environmental health officers and the medical profession. Reliable and valid methods of assessing physical and mental disability are of paramount importance for the success of such a system (the OPCS disability score might be appropriate for the former at least). Housing managers would play the key role in coordinating the system but there would be standard forms for applicants and for letters from GPs. Clear criteria would be specified, based on applicants' handicaps and not on their diseases, and assessment should be a joint process. The actual accommodation proposed would ideally be matched specifically with an individual's needs.

It can be argued that such a system would produce a more effective and integrated response to the needs of those requiring public sector accommodation, including those currently categorized as 'special needs'. Such a system would also, paradoxically, reduce the medicalization of housing need. However even in this ideal model greater consideration would have to be given to issues of equity and evaluation of effectiveness, and the substantial time and resources required for such assessments should not be overlooked (Gardner and Troop 1981).

The rehabilitation paradigm would be the most suitable model for the medical input required in this system. PHPs have no training in rehabilitation and their role in MPR for individuals is therefore inappropriate. Further thought is needed as to who should provide the input from the medical profession. There is currently a shortage of consultants in rehabilitation and it is likely that they would not have the time or perhaps the motivation to become further involved. General practitioners can provide the medical and social context perhaps acting in conjunction with occupational therapy departments and social workers, but they need greater training in the housing process and tighter guidelines about the information required. Conversely, housing officers would benefit from a better understanding of the medical processes underlying many of the handicaps and the evidence relating housing and health.

What, then, should be the role of PHPs? The prime function of public health medicine is to assess the health needs of populations and to evaluate the services provided to meet them. There is a professional interest in preventing disease and promoting health. Given that this paper has argued that there are a range of people in any community who have legitimate health reasons, current or potential, for needing better housing, with or without social support and specific health care interventions, it is clear that PHPs can contribute to an effective approach to housing and health issues. PHPs can work for an intersectoral and integrated approach to defining these groups in relation to current provision, in planning appropriate services and in evaluating the outcomes. This would entail a rethink of the present inflexible 'special needs' housing system and emphasize the fundamental role of housing within the post-Griffiths community care era. PHPs could begin to fulfil a 'health advocacy role', arguing for a housing policy which promotes health for all. This will be increasingly important as the housing crisis deepens still further in the 1990s, with housing inequity widening and housing need growing.

References

Clapham D, Smith S J 1990 Housing policy and 'special needs'. *Policy and Politics* **18**: 193–205

Cole O, Farries J S 1986 Rehousing on Medical grounds—assessment of its effectiveness. *Public Health* **100**:229–35

Commission for Racial Equality 1984 *Race and council housing in Hackney.* Commission for Racial Equality, London

Commission for Racial Equality 1989 *Racial discrimination in Liverpool City Council.* Report of a formal investigation into the housing department. Commission for Racial Equality, London

Davey Smith G, Bartley M, Blane D 1990 The Black report on socioeconomic inequalities in health ten years on. *British Medical Journal* **301**:373–77

Department of the Environment 1988 *Housing trailers to the 1981 and 1984 Labour Force Surveys.* HMSO, London

Department of the Environment 1989a *Housing and construction statistics 1978–1988.* Department of the Environment, Scottish Development Office, Welsh Office, London

Department of the Environment 1989b *Homelessness statistics.* HMSO, London

Donabedian A 1966 Evaluating the quality of medical care. *Millbank Memorial Fund Quarterly* **44**:166–206

Elton P J, Packer J M 1986 A prospective randomised trial of the value of rehousing on the grounds of mental ill-health. *Journal of Chronic Diseases* **39**:221–27

Elton P J, Packer J M 1987 Neurotic Illness as grounds for medical priority for rehousing. *Public Health* **101**:233–42

Faculty of Public Health Medicine (FPHM) 1990a *Survey of Directors of Public Health.* Unpublished findings, Housing and Health Working Party

Faculty of Public Health Medicine (FPHM) 1991 *Housing or homelessness : a public health perspective.* Housing and Health Working Party. FPHM, London

Fisk M J 1982 Medical assessments and priority for housing. *Health Bulletin* **42**:92–96

Gardner PA, Troop PA 1981 Medical priority for rehousing. *Housing* **17**:20–21

Hodgson S 1975 Criteria for rehousing on medical grounds. *Public Health* **90**:15–20

Howells E L 1984 Housing Lines. *British Medical Journal* **288**:201

Kohli H S 1986 Medical housing 'lines'. *British Medical Journal* **293**:370–71

Lalonde M 1984 *A new perspective on the health of Canadians.* Minister of Supply and Services, Ottawa

Llewelyn-Davies H 1990 *Where does the money come from? Grant aid for special needs projects.* SHIL, SITRA, London

Lowry S 1990a Housing and Health. *British Medical Journal* **299**:1261–62

Lowry S 1990b Housing for people with special needs. *British Medical Journal* **300**:321–23

Maclennan W J, Grant J, Forbes B, Urquart J M, Taylor-Brown O 1982 The relevance of health to rehousing in old age. *Health Bulletin* **41**:181–87

Maxwell R J 1984 Quality assessment in health. *British Medical Journal* **288**:1460–72

Morris J N 1990 Inequalities in health: ten years and little further on. *Lancet* (ii):491–93

Muir Gray, Yarnell W G 1979 Housing, health and illness. *Housing* **15**:10–13

Niner P 1989 *Housing needs in the 1990s.* National Federation of Housing Associations, London

Office of Population Censuses and Surveys 1988 *OPCS surveys of disability in Great Britain, Report 1: the prevalence of disability amongst adults*. HMSO, London

Parsons L 1987 Medical priority for rehousing. *Public Health* **101**:435–441

Prescott-Clarke P, Allen P, Morrissey C (Department of the Environment) 1988 *Queueing for Housing: a study of council housing waiting lists*. London, HMSO

Roderick P J, Victor C V, Connelly J B 1991 Is housing a public health issue? A survey of Directors of Public Health. *British Medical Journal* **302**:157–160

Shelter 1990 *Housing briefing paper*. Shelter, London

Smith S J 1990 Health status and the housing system. *Social Science and Medicine* **31**: 753-762

Thomas H F, Yarnell J W G 1978 Housing health and illness. *British Medical Journal* (ii):358–9

World Health Organization 1989 *Health principles of housing*. Geneva, WHO

6 Housing, independent living and physically disabled people

Jenny Morris

'Independent (or Integrated) Living' is part of the international civil rights movement of disabled people. It is a term which describes the aspirations of disabled people in a society which denies them basic human rights. The 1975 United Nations Declaration of Rights of Disabled Persons asserted the right of disabled people to be self-reliant, to live as they choose and to participate in the social, creative and recreational activities of their communities. If disabled people do not have a home which is physically suited to them, together with whatever help they may require to enable them to live in that home, then such basic human rights are unachievable.

In recent years, disabled people and their organizations have identified the ways in which they are being denied the right to their own home. It is clear that the provision of housing across all tenures ignores the physical requirements of disabled people. This, the bricks and mortar part of disabled people's housing needs, is very important. For many disabled people, unwanted dependence on others would disappear overnight if they lived in a physical environment which did not handicap them.

For others, independent living means not just physically suitable housing but also personal assistance to enable them to live in their own home. Our society has generally failed to provide the support services required to enable disabled people to participate in basic human rights: those whose disability is such that they require personal assistance have been consigned either to institutions or to enforced dependence on their families.

Policy makers have assumed for too long that residential care is the most appropriate provision for 'severely disabled' people. Disabled people themselves have demanded more and more that disability must not mean that they should forfeit their right to a home of their own. However, if disabled people are to participate in society on the same basis as non-disabled people neither should they have to depend for their physical care on those with whom they have personal relationships. As one disabled person put it, 'Why should the price of a relationship with me be that of being an unpaid carer?'. It is conceivable that some disabled people may positively choose either residential care or reliance on family members. However, in the current situation of a lack of alternatives, no real choice is possible (Brissenden 1989).

This paper identifies the extent to which local authorities are meeting the need for housing and support services amongst disabled people: highlighting examples of good practice. It is based on a survey carried out on a representative sample of local authority Housing and Social Services Departments in England and Wales. The full research report, *Our Homes Our Rights: Housing, Independent Living and Physically Disabled People* was published by Shelter in 1990.

The paper starts by identifying the important role that local authority housing and social services departments have, and will continue to have, in facilitating independent living for physically disabled people. The second section outlines the survey while the third and fourth sections present the findings with respect to housing and social services departments.

Role of local authorities

Physically disabled people have a number of requirements to enable them to live in their own homes and to fully participate in the life of their community:

1   supply of purpose built or purpose-rehabilitated housing at a reasonable cost;
2   adaptations to existing properties;
3   equipment to maximise independence;
4   personal assistance services are required by some disabled people.

Local authorities' key role in meeting these housing and housing related needs of disabled people partly stems from the lack of economic power which disabled people experience and which means that the private market currently has little to offer them. The OPCS survey found that only 31 per cent of disabled adults under pensionable age are in paid employment and, in the case of around half the disabled adults under pensionable age, there were no earners in the family unit at all (OPCS 1988). Two-thirds of disabled people are over 60 years of age. Disability becomes increasingly common amongst those of 70 and 80 years of age and these people experience a high risk of being on a low income. Poverty is positively correlated with being very old, and this is especially marked for disabled people.

Given their economic disadvantages, it is not surprising that disabled people commonly experience housing disadvantage, nor that they rely disproportionately on council housing. Forty-five per cent of disabled adults are council or housing association tenants compared with 31 per cent of the general population (OPCS 1988, p 12). This situation arises partly because access into the council sector is on the basis of housing need rather than ability to pay. An additional factor is that local authorities have been, and remain, the main providers of wheelchair and mobility accommodation with very little provision in either the housing association, the private rented, or the owner occupied sector.

An important feature of disabled people's access to the housing they require is the increasing difficulty in gaining access to the public rented sector. The rise in the general level of homelessness over the last decade is indicative of the increasing pressure on the declining number of council properties. Disabled people have been disproportionately affected because of their reliance on the public rented sector. They have also been particularly affected by the decline in new build programmes as the housing association and private sectors have not been building wheelchair and mobility accommodation at the rate that local authorities were. The result is that homelessness amongst physically disabled people increased by 92 per cent between 1980 and 1986 compared to 57 per cent amongst all types of household (Morris 1988a).

In the owner-occupied sector, which now accounts for 63 per cent of all households, disabled people are more likely than other households to experience poor housing conditions. This is partly because of the association between old age and poor housing conditions but it is primarily because of the association between poor housing conditions and low income owners. As the English House Condition Survey put it, 'poor housing [is] related, above all, to income' (DoE 1988, p 41).

Local authorities' key role also stems from their legal obligations under the 1970 and 1986 legislation. The evidence is, however, that the extent to which these statutory requirements are fulfilled varies greatly. The Prince of Wales' Advisory Group on Disability, for example, has drawn attention to the problems faced by severely disabled adults below the age of 60. Their report, Living Options Lottery, concluded that:

> the reality of housing and care support options revealed.... is alarming. ....few people obtain the flexible, dependable services essential for personal autonomy. The amount and kind of help a disabled person receives is determined less by need than by chance—a 'living options' lottery (Fiedler 1988).

There are major changes taking place affecting the way in which both housing and social services departments can meet the housing and housing related needs of disabled people. Government policy aims to establish the primacy of the market in the distribution of housing and to limit local authorities' role to an enabling one. Local housing departments are increasingly looking to the private sector and to housing associations to meet the housing needs of their local population. However, it would be foolish to ignore the continuing important role that local authorities have to play as landlords. One in four of all households and about one in two of disabled households are still in the public rented sector. Almost all wheelchair housing and the majority of mobility housing is owned by local authorities.

At the same time, the Government's acceptance of the Griffiths Report on the organization of community care means that local authority social services departments will have an increasingly important role to play in the organization of support services to people in their own homes and of various forms of residential care —even if the social services department is not directly providing the service. Moreover, disabled individuals and their organizations are becoming more aware of both the potential of severely disabled people for independent living and of the inadequacy of the resources and services currently available to make this possible. The British Council of Organisations of Disabled People, local disability organisations and Centres for Independent/Integrated Living are all increasing the pressure on central and local government to provide the necessary housing and support services required to enable disabled people to participate fully in society. This pressure on both housing and social services departments for affordable, suitable housing, with support services where necessary, is likely to increase substantially in the next decade. Local authorities need comprehensive and coherent policies to meet both these demands and their minimum legal obligations, and the research outlined in this paper makes one step in that direction.

A sample of 21 local authorities in England and Wales was taken, using the Department of the Environment's classification of local authority areas to ensure representation across different regions and types of area. Housing and Social Services

Departments were contacted and a questionnaire sent requesting information on:

> knowledge of the need which existed amongst disabled people in their population;
> provision of housing and housing related services;
> details of policies directed at meeting the housing and housing related needs of disabled people.

In addition to the information provided directly by the local authorities, an analysis was carried out of the 1988/89 Housing Investment Programme statements for each authority and of various other statistics collected by the Department of Environment. The number of significantly disabled people in each area was calculated using the OPCS *Disability Survey* and an age and gender breakdown of each area's population. This paper focuses on the responses from the local authorities in the survey; the statistical analysis using the data mentioned above is published in the full research report (Morris 1990).

It should be noted that this survey is based on what the local authorities themselves say about their policies and practices. It may be the case that disabled people's experience of the services provided by local authorities is at variance with the policies which appear in reports, strategy statements, etc. We have, however, felt it useful to name a handful of local authorities who did submit evidence of policies which we felt should be encouraged. This does not mean that these particular local authorities are doing everything right—indeed most of them recognize that they are not. It may also be the case that policies and practices have changed since the survey was carried out, for example because of a change in political control which has occurred in one of the local authorities concerned.

Role of the housing departments

Housing strategies and housing policies

Only three housing departments actually had a written policy on meeting the housing needs of disabled people. In two cases these policies had been developed as a result of dialogue between the housing department and local disability organisations. The policies covered: new build programmes; adaptation of existing stock; modernization programmes; allocation procedures; grants to private owners; staff training.

However, most housing departments had no specific policies on meeting disabled people's housing needs. Very few even mentioned such needs in their housing strategy and when they did there was little to indicate that a strategy really existed. One local housing authority stated in its housing strategy statement that there was 'A need for greater provision of special needs accommodation for the disabled and handicapped', yet there was no indication as to how such accommodation was to be provided. Its detailed strategy concentrated on sheltered housing for elderly people and on housing for single people. There was no indication that, either within its own construction programme of housing for single people or in its collaboration with a local housing association, any consideration was being given to the housing needs of single disabled people.

This exposes a common practice—that of separating out disabled people's housing needs from the rest of the population. If a housing department was developing a strategy on homelessness, there was no recognition that disabled people become homeless as well, and conversely, that some homeless households contain disabled people. Thus, where a council was developing hostel accommodation to cut down on the use of bed and breakfast there was no provision within that hostel accommodation for disabled people. Similarly, a number of housing departments were developing policies aimed at meeting the housing needs of their ethnic minority communities, yet only one such authority explicitly recognized that disabled people would also be part of such communities.

No housing department had a policy on identifying vacant properties with adaptation potential. This is a crucial oversight as, with the reduction in new build programmes, it is often only by adapting existing property that any significant increase in the supply of housing for disabled people can be achieved. The only issue which had been addressed on voids was whether a longer turn round period could be accepted where a property became vacant which had been adapted. Local authority housing departments under pressure to keep down void levels obviously find it difficult to reconcile this with the need to spend some time finding suitable applicants for what are often very individualized adaptations.

The survey did, however, identify one good practice example of integrating disabled people's housing needs into housing strategies. This was Rochdale Metropolitan Borough Council whose housing department appointed a Special Needs Housing Officer who, working with the local disability organisation, developed a comprehensive policy for meeting the housing needs of disabled people. An important part of this policy is the recognition that the housing department has to also concern itself with the support services which are often necessary to enable disabled people to live in their own homes. Yet the department is also aware that disabled people do not want to live in 'special housing schemes' set apart from the rest of the community. As part of the implementation of such a policy, Rochdale has built all new housing to mobility standard since 1980, a significant number to wheelchair standard, and has an expanding capital budget for adaptations to existing stock.

Awareness of housing needs

There was a general impression of a lack of knowledge of housing need amongst disabled people in each local authority area. Information on numbers of elderly and disabled households and of the supply of suitable accommodation, together with adaptations carried out, is provided annually by local authorities to the Department of the Environment, yet the majority of housing departments stated that this information was not available. This paradox is explained by the fact that information about the housing need of disabled people, and the extent to which the local authority is meeting that need, were not part of the operational priorities of most housing departments. Thus the figures may be provided once a year when Government requires them but they are of no relevance to the operation of the housing department throughout the rest of the year. It must also mean of course that the figures provided by the local authority on their HIP returns are highly questionable.

Only three of the housing departments who provided information were able to state how many households on their waiting or transfer list required wheelchair or mobility housing and only two of these were able to break this information down by bedroom size. One housing department responded that they were unable to provide such information 'due to the fact that our computer system under which the Letting system operates does not contain any information on an applicant's (or transfer applicant's) physical disabilities, and so to complete it would entail manually sifting through all of our 3,000 odd applications.' This situation is not uncommon.

Only four local authorities were able to state how many households had been housed into wheelchair or mobility accommodation during the previous year and five were able to say whether any such nominations had been made to housing associations. Again, this lack of information indicates a distinct lack of concern about whether the housing needs of disabled people are being met.

Access to housing

Most housing departments failed to integrate disabled people into their allocation policies. The assumption generally seemed to be that when a disabled person applied for housing they would be referred for medical assessment, usually by the local authority's own Medical Officer. Such a practice has been criticized by disabled people and their organizations as it fails to take account of the practical difficulties of living in unsuitable housing and focuses instead on health problems (though this may vary between authorities). In these circumstances, it is possible for a disabled person's housing need to remain unrecognized.

The failure to integrate disabled people into allocation policies is illustrated by one typical local authority who produced a booklet *A Guide to the Waiting List* which set out the criteria which would qualify a household for rehousing. No mention at all was made of disability. Furthermore, it was clear from the booklet that only households with children, who had no home of their own, and lived in overcrowded conditions, or elderly people needing warden assisted accommodation, had any chance of rehousing. A disabled person living in physically unsuitable housing might assume that there was no point in registering on the waiting list, unless they happened to fall into one of the categories mentioned.

It was also common for housing departments to specifically exclude homeowners from being eligible for rehousing. This can discriminate against disabled owner-occupiers whose property may be totally unsuitable for them. Such a person may be unable to leave hospital or other forms of institutional care, may be made dependent on others, or may be imprisoned within their own home because of the physical characteristics of their house. They may be unable to afford to buy appropriate housing, or in some areas such housing may not exist in the private sector, and thus would look to the local housing authority to solve their housing problem. In most areas, however, the door will be slammed in their face because of the housing department's assumption that owner-occupiers can meet their own housing needs.

A good practice example of incorporating disabled people into an allocations policy was again provided by Rochdale Metropolitan Borough Council. Their points scheme includes a pointing system for a housing problem resulting from disability. The Department's Special Needs Housing Officer has responsibility for determining the level of points. The comprehensive information which is given to all applicants for housing states:

Housing for people with a disability ?
The Council will adapt properties for people with a disability, for example, provision of ramps for wheelchair access, bath, handrails, showers, wider door spaces and, if necessary, an extension to provide bedroom/bathroom facilities at ground floor level. Also, vertical or stair lifts are installed.

Properties have also been purpose build for disabled people.

First of all the Social Services Department's Occupational Therapist will establish whether your present home can be made suitable for you. Where possible this will be done in preference to rehousing.

If the property cannot be adapted the Housing Services Department will try to provide you with a suitable new home which will either be already adapted to the needs of a disabled person, or could be suitably adapted.

Advice and information can be obtained from the Special Needs Officer on (Tel. no.)

Knowledge of supply of dwellings

Five local authority housing departments were able to give information on the numbers of wheelchair and mobility properties in their stock, but only two of these were able to break them down according to bedroom size. Only one authority knew how many such properties were provided by housing associations in their area. There was a similar lack of knowledge on the supply of adapted accommodation. Only two local authorities stated that they held information on adaptations done, although one other thought that this information was possible to get but would require a lot of work. Once again, Rochdale Council was highlighted as a good practice example. Their housing department has a record of all property broken down into the following categories:

1   Purpose built for people with a disability.
2   Adapted with ramps for wheelchair access.
3   Fitted with a lift.
4   Extended for use by a person with a disability.
5   Particularly suited to a person with a disability (due to location, design of property, etc).

This information was also broken down into bedroom size and area. It is therefore possible to identify gaps in supply.

It is difficult to see how a local authority housing department can develop a strategy to meet the housing needs of its disabled population with no proper data on at least the expressed demand and the supply of dwellings within its own housing stock. Ideally, there should be more comprehensive information on housing need and the supply of dwellings across all tenures—particularly if local authorities are to take on more of an enabling role. It is the lack of such information which leads to the common misapprehension that housing for disabled people should be one bedroom properties, whereas the majority of the demand for housing from disabled people below the age of 60 is for two bedroom and above (Robinson 1987; Morris 1986; Morris 1988b).

Adaptation of existing dwellings

Only three local authorities had a specific policy on adaptations to dwellings occupied by disabled council tenants. It was clear that some authorities who did at least have budgetary provision for adaptations treated such expenditure as revenue expenditure when in fact it can be treated as capital expenditure, thus making more money available. Local authority housing departments require a close working relationship with Occupational Therapists employed within the social services departments, who advise on the technical aspects of adaptations. However, some housing departments, who had no specific policy or budget for adaptations to existing council properties, clearly had very little knowledge of the work of Occupational Therapists.

The whole system of grant aid to householders for improvement of dwellings has been changed with the *1990 Housing Act* which introduces means testing, and the Government has now published regulations for determining who is eligible for grant aid. Although the new system has the advantage of abolishing the upper limit for adaptation grants, it remains to be seen whether the operation of a means test will significantly limit the potential for securing adaptations.

Most local authorities increased their expenditure on improvement grants between 1982–84 but expenditure since then has declined. As money has become tighter, adaptation to the housing of disabled and elderly people has often been targeted as a priority within improvement grant programmes. Indeed by 1988 such expenditure accounted for about 40 per cent of all improvement grants nationally and a much higher percentage in some areas. However, in most areas the actual number of adaptations being funded was very small. For example, in one local authority in our survey, only one grant was made in 1987–88 to a disabled private owner. This contrasts with another local authority whose private sector was half the size of the first authority but who gave 91 grants to disabled private owners.

The survey identified Wakefield Metropolitan District Council as providing a good practice example. Their housing department had set up an Adaptations and Disability Unit bringing together staff from Social Services, Environmental Health, and the Housing departments who until then had provided a somewhat fragmented service. The general motivation of the Unit is the recognition that:

People with disabilities require access to information services to assist planning their existing homes or in the organisation of suitable adaptations to enable them to participate fully in the opportunities and challenges of everyday life.

101

The unit deals with private and public sector residents, minor and major adaptations, as well as requests for equipment, and coordinates both the physical carrying out of the work and its financing.

Partnerships with the private sector

There was little indication that local authority housing departments were considering the needs of disabled people when entering into relationships with private developers and housing associations. This was the case even where a local authority had clearly identified the housing needs of various priority groups within its area and had a clearly worked out strategy for enabling these needs to be addressed by the private sector or by housing associations. The focus tends to be on attempting to increase the supply of low cost housing through shared ownership schemes etc but there is no indication that housing authorities are using their relationship with the private sector to encourage building to a broader average, let alone any provision of housing to mobility or wheelchair standards. This is short sighted as such dwellings will be around for at least the next 60 years.

A typical example was that of a rural authority which, having identified the growing number of elderly people as a major source of pressure on its dwindling stock of single storey housing, still failed to identify a need to persuade the private sector to build to mobility standards. This is a significant missed opportunity, for there are many aspects of the local authority's role as enabler—through the provision of land, planning permission and so on—which should make it possible to exert such influence on the private sector. This is particularly the case where the partnership is with a housing association, yet housing association schemes continue to be artificially divided into 'special needs' and 'general needs' housing. Building to a broader average now—on all schemes—will reduce the need for adaptation or the misery of living in unsuitable housing later on.

Liaison between housing and social services departments

Two local authorities reported that they had a formal liaison structure involving housing and social services departments, two others indicating that such formal liaison occurred from time to time. The majority said that liaison was on an informal basis and mainly related to individual cases. (This issue is dealt with in more detail under the analysis of the response of social services departments). There seemed to be little awareness of the way in which the mainstream activities of the housing department—as providers, allocators and landlords of housing—is of relevance to attempts by social services officers to enable independent living for disabled people. For example, one district council's housing department was proud of its support for a Resource Centre, jointly funded with social services, which would 'enable the physically and mentally handicapped to learn life skills'. Yet the housing department had no strategy for providing the accommodation required to enable people to use 'life skills' by living independently.

Social services' response

Knowledge of disabled people and their needs

Local authority social services departments (SSDs) had a greater knowledge of the number of disabled people in their area than did housing departments and were also more likely to have specific policies on meeting their needs. This is not surprising since the legal responsibilities of SSDs, under the *1970 Chronically Sick and Disabled Persons Act* and the *1986 Disabled Persons Act* are more clear cut and physical disability is more clearly established as an area of concern for SSDs. However, the extent of the knowledge and of the policies was still surprisingly inadequate.

For example, the majority of SSDs relied on the *Register of Disabled Persons* for their sole information source on the number of disabled people in the area in spite of the fact that Registers are generally agreed to give gross underestimates. Only three had carried out surveys to estimate the number of physically disabled people amongst their population. One other said that, from time to time 'specialist surveys' were carried out, although none of these gave an adequate overall picture.

Residential care

It was evident from the committee and working party reports which were submitted by a number of the SSDs in the survey that residential care is still considered as inevitable for many disabled people. Sometimes this is viewed as the solution of last resort, forced upon disabled people and those working with them because of a lack of housing and support services. However, more often there seems to be a lack of awareness of either the potential for independent living or of the way in which a denial of independent living is a denial of a basic human right.

When asked whether they knew how many disabled people were in residential care, the majority of SSDs in the survey knew how many were in local authority institutions but only two knew how many were in health authority run facilities, and five how many were in private and voluntary facilities. Only three SSDs said that they did not use residential facilities outside their area. It would appear therefore that the majority of SSDs are placing physically disabled people in residential accommodation outside their own community and have little knowledge about them. This can apply even to disabled children. One local authority admitted that, because it did not have any residential placements inside its boundaries and because it had no fostering or adoption policy for severely disabled children, it was placing severely disabled children, including those under the age of five, 100 miles away or more in residential care.

Role of social services departments in facilitating independent living

Social services departments have two key roles to play in facilitating independent living, namely, working with housing departments to ensure that appropriate accommodation is available; and ensuring that support services are available to disabled people in their own homes. Three SSDs had developed strategies for independent living and three others were in the process of developing such a policy. Additionally, a number of SSDs had obviously given thought to the principles which should motivate their service delivery to disabled people. However, with three exceptions, there was little evidence that disabled people and their organizations were properly consulted about the kind of service which they wanted.

Derbyshire County Council has long been a good practice example in terms of their *Principles of Service Delivery*. Their social services department, which has been working with organizations of disabled people for the last ten years, adopted the following general aim in their *Strategic Plan* in 1983:

> To secure independent, integrated living opportunities for disabled people in order to promote their full participation in the mainstream of economic, social and political life.

The following service principles were then developed:

> Services aiming to restore, sustain or enhance value and dignity for people who need our help should:

104

1   be based on an assessment of what these people want and need, and what most people approve and prefer;
2   be local so that people are not removed from their homes or community unless they so choose;
3   support and supplement existing positive personal and social relationships;
4   provide shelter based on ordinary domestic arrangements;
5   be comprehensive so that the needs of people are met across a very wide area of their lives in coordinated and continuous ways;
6   impose no restrictions beyond those compatible with each individual's readiness to grow in ability, independence and self-determination.

A number of SSDs mentioned that statutory work with children had increased so much during recent years that social workers had little time for other client groups. A lack of knowledge and training in the area of physical disability was also identified.

Working with housing departments

There was little evidence of housing and social services departments working together to facilitate independent living. Most SSDs had a history of working closely with health authorities through Joint Care Planning Teams (JCPTs) (which coordinate joint projects and funding for common client groups of health and social services) but these often did not include representatives from the local authority housing department(s). Some JCPTs have held policy seminars and conferences in the last few years on services for disabled people and sometimes significant policy initiatives have developed in this type of forum. However, it is apparent that when initial policy discussions are held it is rare for the relevant housing department(s) to be represented. This is either because SSDs and health authorities have failed to identify the role of housing officers, or because when they have, housing departments have failed to respond. The latter situation is particularly likely to arise when there is no one housing officer with responsibility for physical disability.

Where a local authority had started to develop and implement policies aimed at meeting the housing needs of disabled people, the initiatives usually involved *either* the housing department *or* the social services department, but rarely both. Thus it was common for housing departments to complain that SSDs were not playing their full part in, for instance, offering technical advice on adaptations, or in providing personal assistance support within the home. In turn, SSDs often despaired of being able to find suitable accommodation for physically disabled people and complained that housing officers made unwarranted assumptions about the inability of disabled people to live independently. One social services department, for example, had great difficulty in persuading a district council housing department to offer accommodation to a single mother who became disabled and who wished to leave hospital to set up home again and look after her daughter.

Although it may be assumed that the split between social services functions on a county level and housing functions on a district council level may make it more difficult for the departments to work together, coterminous boundaries did not seem to make it any more likely that social services and housing departments would be working closely together.

The survey identified one local authority which was developing good practice in the area of coordination between housing and social services departments. This was Kensington and Chelsea Borough Council whose SSD has set up a formal working party of housing and social services representatives 'to facilitate better planning of services between the two departments'. However, this type of cooperation is only possible when both departments have specialist officers covering physical disability and it is clear that this local authority has much development work to do.

Dorset county council SSD had set up a working party on 'The Accommodation Needs of Physically Handicapped Clients', and had identified a range of requirements—from full residential care to independent accommodation. Unfortunately, their survey of the accommodation needs of disabled people relied on social workers' and occupational therapists' assessments and the membership of the working party did not include representation from disabled people. However, the report included a useful identification of the way in which the SSD should encourage the provision of more appropriate accommodation. Under the heading of *Meeting the Needs for Independent Accommodation* the following recommendations were made:

1 Both local authorities and the Housing Corporation should be made aware of the shortage of suitable accommodation for disabled people in Dorset.

2 Local housing authorities should be made aware of the positive results of the Christchurch Charter for Disabled People, and should be encouraged to adopt their own similar Charters.

3 The maintenance of records of properties suitable for disabled people, to include both mobility housing and wheelchair housing, would be helpful. At present not every housing authority is able to identify which or how many of its own stock is adapted for disabled people. This question could be pursued both locally and nationally.

4   The department should contribute to structure plans, town and village plans and other planning consultation documents by specifying the need for:

   a all houses to have a downstairs toilet and one room downstairs which could become a bedroom;

   b all ground floor accommodation to be built to mobility standards

   c at least a small percentage of all new ground floor accommodation to be built to wheelchair standards.

5   The advantages of the adoption of such policies by planning authorities and housing authorities would include not only readier access to housing for disabled people, but also an increasing saving on the cost to local and county departments of funding adaptations for disabled clients.

Provision of support services

Only three SSDs had a strategy for helping disabled people to achieve independent living. Three other authorities were currently preparing such a strategy. The majority of authorities had no 'personal care packages' for individual clients, relying instead on *ad hoc* arrangements, mainly consisting of utilising the Home Care service (home helps). Only two authorities actually had a separate budgetary provision for personal care packages. One was a rural authority and funded 10 disabled clients' personal care needs. In contrast, an urban authority—with a much larger population—was considering funding two clients. This is the 'lottery' which the Prince of Wales Advisory Group's report was referring to. Whether someone can live independently depends so much on where they live and whether their local authority has recognized the need for an independent living strategy for disabled people.

Two of the departments who are in the process of developing independent living strategies already provide some support. One employs 12 care assistants, whose services are provided free to physically disabled clients. One other authority has a joint budget with the health authority which uses Crossroads Care Attendant Scheme (a national voluntary organization providing care attendants) and health care assistants (funded by the health authority).

Transition to independent living

For some disabled people their experience of dependence makes independence difficult to achieve. Someone who has been in residential care for a number of years, for example, may find independent living an initially frightening prospect. Younger disabled people are often denied the experiences which enable them to become adults independent of their parents.

Some SSDs have identified the need for strategies to aid the transition to independent living although unfortunately it is more common to expect the disabled person to find all the motivation within themselves. The four SSDs in the survey who had developed projects which attempt to provide a transition to independent living had either successfully cooperated with the housing authority to provide accommodation or had made provision out of their own capital budget. In another area, a local voluntary organization had attempted to set up a project aimed at young disabled people living with their parents but the scheme foundered when the Housing Corporation refused funding for the accommodation involved.

Any such scheme must also plan for permanent accommodation and personal assistance and indeed it was the difficult experience of getting district councils within their area to house people who had tried out the transition project and wanted to live independently which prompted one social services department to address themselves to their role in influencing local housing authorities.

Dorset county council SSD has developed a scheme which the survey identified as a good practice example in aiding the transition to independent living. This scheme enables disabled people who have been in institutional care or young people living with their parents to try out living independently. Two flats were provided, one to mobility, the other to wheelchair standard, and personal assistance provided through the home help service and a care attendant scheme. When an assessment was made of the operation of the scheme, it was found that some of the users felt the professional assessment of their ability to live independently was intrusive. This is potentially a drawback of any such scheme in that it can turn into a 'test' for disabled people where non-disabled professionals judge them. However, this particular SSD recognised the dangers of this and decided that in future professional assessments would only be done at the client's request, in order to recommend ways of coping or to provide a professional report to accompany a housing application.

The scheme was found to be particularly useful for younger disabled people living with their parents:

> Fieldwork staff.... felt that change would not have been possible without the use of [the scheme] to boost confidence and prove the client's capabilities. Indeed, the clients and their social workers feel that the question [of leaving the parental home] may not even have arisen.

Working with disabled people and their organizations

The majority of SSDs participated in a JCPT (with health authorities) for disabled people and the majority included representatives from disabled people's organizations. However, it was clear that many of the organizations represented were those run by non-disabled people *for* disabled people rather than from organizations *of* disabled people.

Again Derbyshire county council SSD provides the good practice example of involving disabled people in the development and implementation of policy. For some years the SSD has funded a Centre for Integrated Living (CIL) which is run by disabled people and staffed mainly by disabled people. Its role is to develop, together with the local authority, initiatives which would aid independent living. It also acts as an important source of information for disabled people, acting as advocates where necessary. The local authority has continued to respond to new roles as they were identified, for example, by funding the CIL to maintain a register of adapted housing in the district.

Conclusion

The picture which emerges from the survey is a grim one for disabled people. They look to local authority housing and social services departments to help them achieve a basic human right. A lucky few live in parts of the country where their local authority will be able to respond with the housing and support services that they need to live independently. The majority, however, will find that there is little knowledge of the needs of the physically disabled community; that there are no policies for meeting such needs; and that housing and social services departments are failing to work together to help disabled people achieve the things which most non-disabled citizens take for granted.

Not only is there a failure to work together at local level, but central government is also failing to provide the legislative and subsidy framework to enable housing and social services departments to jointly address the aspirations of disabled people. The White Paper *Caring for People* and the 1990 legislation which followed recognised that local authority social services departments have a key role to play in enabling disabled people to exert control over their living situations. However, national housing policy continues to be dominated by the promotion of market forces and since 1979 the main policy aim has been a restructuring of tenure rather than the addressing of housing need. Both legislation and public subsidies have been directed at an increase in owner-occupation and an attack on council housing. Such policies have been directly against the interests of disabled people whose economic position and need for housing with particular physical characteristics mean that the private sector has little to offer.

While Government policy fails to link housing policy to other social policy areas, local government fails to integrate disabled people's housing needs into their mainstream activities, and housing and social services departments fail to work together, disabled people will continue to be condemned to institutional care or imprisoned in housing which unnecessarily restricts their lives.

References

Brisenden S 1989 *A charter for personal care* Progress 16 Disablement Income Group, Summer

British Council of Organisations of Disabled People 1987 *Disabled people looking at housing* Report of BCODP's National Housing Conference. (BCODP is the British wing of Disabled People's International)

Department of the Environment 1988 *English house condition survey.* HMSO, London

Fiedler B 1988 *Living options lottery - housing and support services for people with severe physical disabilities.* Prince of Wales Advisory group on Disability, London

Morris J 1986 Housing disabled people—providing for us all, *Housing* November.

Morris J 1988a *Freedom to lose - housing policy and people with disabilities.* Shelter, London

Morris J 1988b *Housing and disabled people in Tower Hamlets.* Action for Disability, London Borough of Tower Hamlets

Morris J 1990 *Our homes, our rights: Housing, independent living and disabled people.* Shelter, London

Office of Population Censuses and Surveys 1988a *Surveys of disability in Great Britain (Report 1, the prevalence of disability among adults)* HMSO,London

Office of Population, Censuses and Surveys 1988b *Surveys of disability in Great Britain (Report 2, the financial circumstances of disabled adults living in private households).* HMSO, London

Robinson I 1987 *Re-evaluating housing for people with disabilities in Hammersmith and Fulham.* London Borough of Hammersmith and Fulham Special Needs Unit

7 AIDS and HIV—a barium meal for the housing system

Roz Pendlebury and Peter Molyneux

Housing and health

It has long been taken for granted that housing has a major influence on public health. Florence Nightingale said that 'the connection between health and the dwellings of the population is one of the most important that exists'. However, when it comes to translating this into action or any expression of housing rights it is a case that has to be continually argued. The housing needs of people with AIDS are no exception.

If we look at a typical list of housing factors associated with ill health there would not necessarily be anything controversial on it. There is a clear relationship between damp and health; there is some recognition of a connection between stairs and mobility. There is a wealth of information to show that deprivation is closely associated with physical ill health, at least as measured by premature mortality. We can show in relation to homelessness and the growth in the use of bed and breakfast accommodation that this has an adverse effect on the health of mothers and babies, both physically and in terms of low level mental illness. However, it is much more difficult to show exactly what effect income, social network, transport and housing have. 'We have a sort of twentieth century miasmatic theory of mental health but there is no sign yet of respectable scientific proof of pathogenesis which would legitimize political action' (Morton 1988).

Even in relation to physical conditions it is relatively easy to show that by improving someone's housing conditions you are improving their wellbeing. It is much more difficult to show that a concerted programme of home improvements for people with

111

HIV will actually improve their life expectancy. We can see that poor housing conditions are a bad thing and that people who are ill will find them harder to deal with but that is seldom enough in the cut throat battle for scarce resources.

There has been a considerable increase in the number of medical priority referrals as the housing situation has deteriorated, even in areas where housing has traditionally been of good quality and in good supply. In studies of new towns with a history of readily available decent housing, demand has outstripped supply as young people and newly married couples have wanted to move away from the parental home. Here there is a corresponding increase in applications on the grounds of mental health from those with an uncertain grip on the housing ladder. People who feel that they would be unlikely to get housed from the waiting list will be keen to maximise any points they have. One way of doing this is through laying greater emphasis on the stress and mental strain caused by overcrowding and poor housing conditions. Obviously this puts pressure on medical practitioners too. As:

> It is crucially important that the consultant undertaking these assessments has some understanding of the housing resources available to the council in order to maintain some degree of reality in the expectations of those seeking priority (Hawes 1989)

The difficulty that also faces the medical practitioner is in assessing the validity of any symptoms in a context where the housing environment is a key element. There have been instances of medical practitioners refusing to recommend transfers for people with HIV on the grounds of mobility since this is purely a housing design matter and not a **medical** need. As with any assessment of medical priority which is affected by perceptions of the housing market, it is also open to being influenced by prejudice and other factors affecting the evaluation of what makes a deserving case. People with HIV have particularly suffered in this respect.

Experience of people with HIV seeking housing

When people with AIDS first started coming forward for housing it was said that they were not the 'sort of people' that priority channels were intended for. Lack of information about transmission of the virus was used as an excuse for witholding a service. Also the refusal of many medical practitioners to treat patients with HIV gave a very clear lead to housing authorities. Medical misinformation was muddled with morals. As one DHA manager said:

Why should we act responsibly when people with HIV didn't
(Raynsford and Morris Consultants, 1989).

Of course the idea of the deserving and undeserving poor is not
new. From the *Artisans' Dwellings Acts* of the 1880s to the
Housing Acts of the 1980s the providers of local authority
housing have struggled with the purpose of such housing and the
extent to which housing management and quality of housing
should be linked to social control (Smith 1990).

There is also the question of what housing is really for. Is it
somewhere for a person to live? Or is it somewhere for a client to
receive services? In 1985 at the Department of Health and Social
Security Conference 'Caring for People with AIDS in the
Community', Michael Adler, Professor of Genitourinary medicine at
the Middlesex Hospital, spoke of the need for hostels for people
with AIDS where equipment could be stored and nursing care more
easily provided. One London DHA was insistent that there were
cost advantages to clustering people. What was puzzling was that
the neighbouring district saw no cost advantages since people were
rarely ill at the same time when not in need of acute services.
Certainly, many community based health professionals spoke solely
of the need for residential care facilities in terms of ease of service
provision and not in terms of how it might feel to live there.

There are still assumptions made about the extent to which
people with AIDS will make demands on housing services. It was
quite common as recently as 1988 to hear doctors talk of their
patients being white middle class gay men who were home owners
and comfortably housed. But these men did not necessarily find that
their homes remained appropriate nor that they could retain a level
of income which was necessary to stay in this type of housing.
Clearly as perceptions of HIV have changed, there has been an
increasing recognition of its effects on working class gay men and
drug users, and on issues such as race, sex, and sexuality as barriers
to housing. Nevertheless, the prejudice remains that people with
HIV are all young and single, and whilst people with HIV may get
themselves housed, this prejudice is frequently reflected in allocation.
From this we can see that in a very short space of time a highly
professionalized view has developed of the needs of people with
HIV and AIDS and it has operated without any clear reference to
what they themselves want (see Jeffrey and Popplestone 1988).

Consumer view

Given this background it was clearly a priority to establish the
'consumer viewpoint'. We established, therefore, two projects.
One was to survey the tenants of the specialist housing schemes

Table 7.1. *Where people were living:*

	%
	%
Owner occupied	19
Local authority	48
Housing association	19
Private rented	9
Other	5
Total	100

Source: Drake (1990) p7

for people with HIV and AIDS, and the other was to ask people with HIV and AIDS what they wanted from their housing. This research was undertaken for the AIDS and Housing Project and The Landmark by Madeleine Drake 1990).

We decided to look at south London because we felt there was a different profile in terms of gender, race and class than in west London where a comparative survey was being carried out by the Royal Borough of Kensington and Chelsea. Also there was likely to be a different housing market in this area. We spent some time discussing the best way of including the broadest range of people possible. In the end we decided that for the pilot we would use clients of clinics and social workers in hospitals. Although we were concerned that people such as refugees might be excluded from these services, they seemed the most value-free point of access available.

This project was seen as a pilot for a larger national survey. We interviewed 50 people over a four week period in July and August 1989. Obviously, this is a small sample, a factor which should be borne in mind when evaluating the findings. It is not possible to present the detailed results here, but there are a number of points of particular interest.

The figures for owner-occupation and the private rented sector in Table 7.1 are typical for this part of London. What would be interesting to look at in more detail is how people achieved access to local authority and housing association stock. Certainly a number of people who had been housed since their diagnosis felt that insufficient attention had been paid to their needs, and most in this category had been housed through hard-to-let schemes. Thus, many of the interviewees felt that they wanted to move, or to adapt their property.

Table 7.2 shows a very high level of dissatisfaction amongst respondents with their housing situation. None of the owner-

Table 7.2.   *Whether people wanted to stay or move*

	%
Move	54
Stay and adapt	29
Stay	17
Total	100

occupiers wanted to move. Those who did want to move, or who wanted adaptations made to their homes, produced a list of requirements that are more an indictment of the standard of housing generally available than a reflection of the lack of fulfilment of specialized needs (Table 7.3).

Many respondents said that they found their accommodation difficult and/or expensive to heat and most of those who were in local authority housing were dependent on portable sources of heat. Many people found bathing difficult or painful and wanted showers, if possible one without a trough. Security was an issue, with several of the interviewees talking about severe harassment. The need to do extra laundry, particularly as a result of night-sweats or diarrhoea, meant that a high proportion of people wanted their own washing and drying facilities. Noise was quoted as an issue for many people and this is one reason for such a high proportion wanting double glazing: heat insulation being the other. In the sample only 9 per cent needed wheelchair access or a stair lift. However, these may be needed by people later on. The main issue here is that people do not want to live with these adaptations until they need them.

From this we can see that the majority of people want access to good quality mainstream housing, suitably adapted, provided that they have adequate support, and that sufficient thought is given to their future needs. As one respondent said:

> I would like to be able to talk with people who understand my condition, to be able to talk with people and relate, rather than be isolated (AIDS and Housing Project and The Landmark, 1990).

However, many respondents expressed a fear that support agencies could not be flexible enough and wondered whether grouped or clustered housing would make this better (Table 7.4). Others were concerned about neighbours and felt that there would be greater security offered by knowing that their neighbours also had HIV.

Table 7.3.   *Requirements of would be movers and adapters*

	%
Central heating	90
Shower	67
Door/window locks	57
Laundry facilities	48
Separate WC	43
Entry phone	43
Double glazing	38
Ground floor accommodation	33
Central alarm	24
Stair lift	9
Wheelchair access	9

Source: Drake (1990) p15

Commenting generally on how their housing affected their health, respondents mentioned how difficult it was to stay well in their accommodation. Some respondents mentioned how long it took to get rehoused and others noted the need to educate the general public and local authorities so that people with HIV infection could remain integrated in the community.

Clearly the message is that most people can be housed through relets provided that the necessary equipment and adaptations can be made quickly. It is important to ensure that there is adequate space for carers, that the bathrooms are large enough—initial feedback from the tenants of specialist schemes for people with HIV is that the bathrooms are invariably too small—and that there is adequate sound proofing. These requirements are all difficult to ensure in existing stock and difficult to fund in new developments. Nevertheless they are achievable. What is also evident is that HIV is as much a management issue as it is a development issue.

Housing management

The main problems facing housing organisations wanting to make stock available to people with HIV are the review internal policies, the difficulty of overcoming fears about infection, and the need to overcome prejudice.

Table 7.4. *What type of housing people wanted to move to*

	per cent
Separate self-contained	55
Grouped self-contained	41
Shared	4

Source: Drake (1990) p13

> The policy issues raised demand a review of existing policies, highlight the lack of policy in other areas and raise questions about housing priority and allocation and resources (AIDS and Housing Project and the National Federation of Housing Associations, 1989).

This is what we refer to as the 'Barium Meal' effect, that is, the point that HIV shows up weaknesses in the housing system that have always been there. This is reflected in the range of guidelines now becoming available (AIDS and Housing Group, Scotland 1989; AIDS and Housing Project and AHG Scotland 1990; Local Authorities Associations' Officer Working Group on AIDS 1988)

Housing providers have had to review their internal policies on infection control, confidentiality (both disclosure and record-keeping), allocations and referrals, equal opportunities and so on. In many cases it is the first time that these issues have been discussed. HIV can also point to inadequacies in the implementation of existing policies—as one housing manager said to us in a training session 'I'm not worried about AIDS, I never go into poof's flats anyway'.

People are often better informed about HIV than other infections such as hepatitis or tuberculosis, but they still come up with a long list of 'what if's', from 'what if the doctors are wrong' to 'what if someone with HIV bites me'. There is also the easy connection between HIV and morality, and the way in which racist, sexist, and heterosexist attitudes inform this relationship. Add to this assumptions about drug users being unreliable tenants and you have a heady mix. All of this counts against people with HIV when housing allocation officers are making hard decisions about who gets what from a list that includes elderly people, people with mental illness, and people with disabilities.

Development

Even where there has been a willingness to act progress has been slow. HIV raises issues that cannot be avoided and which take

117

time to work through. It is hardly surprising then that one response to this slow progress has been to set up specialist housing agencies. Agencies such as Strutton Housing Association and Supported Accommodation Team AIDS—Lothian, by providing flexible management and support, have attempted to create an AIDS educated environment where tenants can be confident that their needs will be properly met and where sensitive, confidential services can be offered.

The Housing Corporation has been keen to see housing associations involved in this area. Its *Circular number 40* published in 1987 was concerned with AIDS. In addition, Scottish Homes supported the publication of *Housing and HIV Disease*. Nevertheless, in the period 1989–90 the development programme could only yield 47 new units nationally and this figure is unlikely to increase. The Department of Environment has thus far refused to make any specific allocation either to the Housing Corporation or through the Housing Investment Programme to local authorities.

It is clear, then, that whilst housing associations provide a few innovative, good quality schemes, it is local authorities who are likely to continue to be the major providers of housing to people with HIV. The Local Authorities Associations recognise this in their guidelines :

> Housing authorities have an overt responsibility both to provide and develop their services for people affected by HIV.... and to respond to the needs of employees, both those directly and those indirectly affected by HIV infection. (Local Authorities Associations' Officer Working Group in AIDS, 1988).

Nevertheless, there is still a lot of work needed on the ground to ensure that policies are implemented and that someone with HIV can walk into their local housing aid centre confident of a sympathetic response.

Conclusion

The 1990 *NHS and Community Care Act* and current reviews of homelessness legislation are ensuring that housing and health are back at the top of the social policy agenda. Yet all too often the housing element in needs assessment is ignored or the existence of appropriate housing is assumed. At a Department of Health and Social Service Conference in 1985 Norman Fowler said 'We must ensure that people with AIDS are able to live and die in their own homes'. Yet in a speech to the House of Commons in 1989 Kenneth Clarke said 'I see no connection between what I am talking about today [Community Care] and housing finance'. We must ensure that there is recognition that housing is a basic human right, and not a commodity to provide a source of investment for the upwardly mobile.

References

AIDS and Housing Group (Scotland) 1990 *Positive housing:* AHG, Glasgow

AIDS and Housing Project and The AIDS and Housing Group (Scotland) 1990 *Housing and HIV disease: policy guidelines for Scottish housing associations.* AHP, London

AIDS and Housing Project and the National Federation of Housing Associations 1989 *Housing and HIV disease: guidelines for housing association action.* NFHA, London

Drake M 1990 *Housing and HIV in south London.* AIDS and Housing Project and The Landmark

Hawes D 1989 Environmental Neurosis. *Housing Review,* 38, July/Aug

Jeffrey R, Popplestone G 1988 Housing advice for people with AIDS *Roof,* March/April, 38–41

Local authorities Associations' Officer Working Group on AIDS 1988 *Housing and HIV infection* Association of Metropolitan Authorities, London

Morton S 1988 All around the houses: Is there any consensus on the major public health problems of housing in the UK? *Radical Community Medicine,* **33**: 3–8

Raynsford and Morris Consultants 1989 *Housing is an AIDS issue.* National AIDS Trust, London

Smith S J 1990 AIDS, Housing and Health *British Medical Journal* **300**: 243–4

8 Accommodation plus support

Paul Spicker

Introduction

There is considerable vagueness about the nature of 'community care', both in theory and in practice. Bayley (1973) makes the important distinction between care 'in' the community—that is, care within an identifiable geographical area—and care 'by the community', which depends on the idea of a community as a network of social relationships. Within this, there are further subdivisions; in *Social Housing and the Social Services,* (1989) I outlined six. Care 'in' the community might be seen as care that is not in an institution, and it can be interpreted as a reaction to the problems of institutional care. It may refer to care in ordinary housing (in France, 'community care' is referred to as *'le maintien à domicile',* which at least has the virtue of honesty), or, more positively, to 'normalization', which implies the fostering of independence, normal social roles, and a degree of risk. Care 'by' the community might be seen as care through those social relationships—an ideal which seems impossibly romantic; care by community–based services; and care by informal carers, who are principally members of the family, and principally women. The meanings of 'community care' are, then, varied and inconsistent.

Despite this inconsistency, the idea of 'community care' has been increasingly influential in shaping the planning of services for different client groups. Community care has come to be associated, after Bayley, with the idea that care can be developed in terms of a range of provisions from which it is possible to construct an individually tailored package of services. The problem with this in practice is that the type of service which is likely to be available does not necessarily conform to the pattern of flexible, responsive options. On one hand, there is a range of conventional services, including housing, social security, education and primary health care, which were devised for the needs of the general population and require major development in order to respond adequately to the specialized and complex needs of the principal client groups needing 'community care'. On the other hand, there are residential units, which often possess specialized skills and developed facilities, but which have been associated with serious problem: they tend to be expensive, inflexible, and socially isolated.

If any government really wanted to move towards the development of community care, they would be wise to start from somewhere else. It is possible to imagine an ideal situation in which there is no 'residential' care in the currently understood sense of the term, in which each person receives a level of care in ordinary housing, wholly divorced from a residential unit, on the lines of 'staying put'. But for this to be practised generally, it would be necessary to have a different kind of organization of care, devoted to the development of peripatetic and domiciliary services; a different pattern of funding; different training, and new professional specialisms; the closure of existing units of residential care; and the guarantee that no one would be discharged from residential institutions without having direct access to ordinary housing of a suitable type and in a suitable location. Somehow, and despite the reforms currently on offer (which seem to me to be about different things entirely), this has an unreal air, and I doubt it is worth spending time discussing the possibility. David Anderson, writing about community care, comments that people seem very happy to spend time talking about spaceships when what we actually need is a bus ride (Anderson, 1981).

The Wagner report

A way forward is offered by the Wagner report on residential care (1988). Wagner seeks to redefine residential care in terms which embrace special housing initiatives, elements of provision which are more usually seen as a form of 'community' care. Residential care has been seen, traditionally, as a type of care diametrically opposed to community care, and residential institutions have been as distinct communities in themselves, set apart from the rest of society. This picture, Wagner argues, is potentially misleading. There are many different types of residential care. They include, for example:

Long term care.	This is the most commonly recognised pattern, including many old people's homes, children's homes, and so on.
Respite care.	This is intended to give carers a break.
Assessment.	A number of homes, particularly for children, are designed as temporary stages, during which a person's needs can be assessed and a suitable placement found.

Rehabilitation.	Some homes, like probation hostels or hostels for former psychiatric patients, are concerned with enabling someone to return to the community.
Therapy or treatment.	Examples are hostels for people with drug dependencies, and some hostels for mentally ill people.
Training.	There are homes and hostels of this type, for example, those for mentally handicapped people, and mothers with young children.
Convalescence.	Examples are, nursing homes for the elderly or for some psychiatric patients.
Crisis or emergencies.	These include shelters and refuges.
Shared care or flexible care.	Arrangements for these needs are increasingly being made for elderly or physically disabled people. (Wagner, 1988, p 166)

The report argues that, in practice, there is no clear distinction to be made between the different forms of care. Residential care should be seen not as care that is different in kind from other types of provision but as a pattern of care provided with accommodation. It is a form of 'supported housing', or 'accommodation plus support'. The report includes, as a result, examples such as sheltered housing and group living or core and cluster homes, as forms of 'residential care', and the review of research even goes so far as to treat arrangements for boarding out as 'residential'. Potentially, the range of services which might be included within this approach is limitless; there is not so much a division between particular types of accommodation, as different levels and types of supportive provision which can be associated for various purposes with a range of different kinds of housing. Residential care, then, fits into the range of options which might be available for the support of people in the community.

There are a number of advantages in this approach. Wagner was seeking to break down the distinction between residential and community care, a distinction which has had undesirable effects in separating residential care from the rest of the community. The problems of residential care have included the development of patterns of living which are in many ways abnormal; the isolation of institutions has fostered practices which deny residents an opportunity for a decent life. The long line of scandals in institutions illustrates the extent to which residents—and staff—are dehumanised through lack of contact with the standards of the world outside (See Martin, 1984), but this situation represents an extreme. The loss of contact with the outside world is more likely to mean that the institution is a 'warehouse' for people in whom society has lost interest.

From the point of view of the residents, the separation of

'accommodation' from 'support' strengthens their position considerably. 'Tenants' have greater rights than 'residents'. A conditional right is necessarily weaker than an unconditional one, and if the right to accommodation is dependent on a person's need for support, it is diminished by it. Wagner's arguments for greater choice depend to a large degree on the possibility that alternative arrangements can be made in other settings.

Treating 'support' as a variable factor means that residents can receive a degree of care tailored to their particular circumstances. The needs of residents vary, and they change over time; consequently, they require a differentiated response. The development of flexible responses makes it possible to provide an increased level of care in a place where a person is settled—for example, nursing care for an old person whose health is deteriorating—or to adapt care to the changing needs of the resident population, such as a group of people with mental handicaps growing older. It is in the nature of many kinds of support, particularly those kinds offered to groups of people whose personal needs fluctuate over time, like elderly people and psychiatric patients, that there will be some uncertainty about the level of need which ought to be provided for. One may feel that people should be offered the minimum amount of support possible, to foster independence—the position usually taken with psychiatric patients. Alternatively, it may be that greater potential support should be offered than is currently required, either in the belief that dependency will increase (the position with elderly people), or because future problems may arise (services for adolescents leaving care).

One of the largest obstacles to appropriate provision is that residential schemes provided for different groups are conceived and produced, not as a range of separate services, but as a whole. If clients do not need the particular services offered within a residential establishment, they should transfer somewhere else. This is easier said than done, partly because the criteria for admission and discharge vary from one service to another, partly because transfer often involves a shift in financial responsibilities, and often because all the appropriate alternative places are full. Elderly people may be provided with residential care in a geriatric ward in hospital, under the remit of the NHS; in private nursing care, currently principally funded by the Department of Social Security, but soon to be the responsibility of Social Services and Social Work departments; in local authority residential care, at regional or county level; in sheltered housing, which is usually administered by district councils or housing associations; or in ordinary housing. If, instead of thinking of each of these options as exclusive of the others, supportive services were treated as being flexible within these different residential settings, there would be scope to adjust the degree of support without requiring a person to move, or falling foul of the problems of moving a person entirely from the responsibility of one service to another. The best example of such arrangements in practice is the growth of 'category $2\frac{1}{2}$', sheltered housing for frail elderly people, often negotiated between housing associations and social services, which straddles the divide between category 2 sheltered accommodation and (in England) part III residential accommodation.

The case against the distinction of accommodation and support

The Wagner report's arguments are powerful, and they carry conviction. At the same time, there are some serious practical problems with the approach which Wagner advocates. There are important differences between services provided to someone within ordinary housing, and services which are only delivered in practice within a specially designated residential setting.The recent white paper refers to community care as including care in 'homely' settings (Cm 849, 1989); but 'homely' settings are not the same as people's homes. People move into special forms of housing primarily because of the kind of support they will be receiving, and this is enough in itself to produce the range of problems associated with residential care. The division of accommodation and support is simply unrealistic; it does not reflect the pattern of services either as they exist, or as they need to exist within current constraints.

In general, residents have some special needs; that is, some characteristics which distinguish them from other people in the population. The populations in different kinds of residential care differ because the needs which are catered for by each type of unit are different. Elderly people in nursing care have a different range of capacities from elderly people in local authority residential homes. Mentally ill people in staffed hostels tend to have a higher level of needs (and usually of dependency) than those in cluster housing. This is not invariably true, but where it is not it is usually because the people are in the wrong places, or in the only places available.

Clapham and Smith (1990) have argued that the designation of 'special needs' is stigmatizing. This is probably true if the population which is served by the residential unit is a stigmatized group, which is the case for many of the clients of special housing initiatives, then the unit is likely to have an associated stigma, exacerbated because the services are being provided within an tifiable physical location. On the face of it, the separation of 'accommodation' from 'support' might help to avoid this, because it is the combination of the two which has fostered the problems of residential care. But the separation is based only on a theoretical distinction, not a practical one. It is evident that services are being provided within an identifiable physical location; the stigma of residential care stems from this basic fact, and it is not necessarily avoided by pretending that one is doing something else. The consequences of not providing the resources are worse.

The importance of the designation of 'special needs' is that it provides a key to access to essential services. Meteyard (1985) argues that there are likely to be problems from denying the special status of residential care. He condemns old people's homes which are designed in imitation of one-star seaside hotels when the needs of frail elderly people demand an environment adapted to their capacities. He argues for the use of large signposts and Tannoy systems, if that is what is needed to help people live with a greater capacity for self-direction. (There are, of course, more subtle ways of achieving similar aims, like colour coding doors and using standard kinds of sign, but the point is nonetheless relevant for that.) In attempting to avoid the destructive elements of the distinction between residential and community care, there is always a risk of ignoring the positive advantages of residential settings for enabling and empowering residents.

Residential care is not like a home in the community. The recipients of residential care have to move into territory which is not theirs to define: it is different by virtue of that alone. Sheltered housing for elderly people has offered the main exception, because within sheltered housing units people are able to decorate as they please, to choose their own furniture, and to fix things on the walls. This offers a model for other kinds of development. But there must be some limitations, partly because of the desire to respond to the needs of the people for whom the service has been developed, such as people who are resident for relatively short periods and people with considerable physical needs and partly because of the logistical problems of administering a unit with staff, an office, different mechanisms of support, and so forth. (There are equally some advantages: one of the bonuses of group living is that one can afford joint leisure facilities, like a games room or library, which are not realistically possible for most people in individual homes.)

Because support is organized in relation to accommodation there is an identifiable pattern of services associated with particular residential units. The capacities of staff have to be developed in relation to the needs of the intended residents. This creates difficulties, because the range of abilities of any single profession is limited, and probably more limited than the very general level of competence required for the production of residential care. Residential work has gradually been established as a form of generic social work, requiring the full range of skills demanded of social workers elsewhere, including not only interviewing, communication, and assessment, but often relatively specialized skills like groupwork. Perversely, the trend to 'genericism' in social work leads in the residential context to a reduced field of activity; the 'generic' approach is generic within social work, not within the range of needs of a particular client group. Other kinds of population require, and receive, different kinds of professional care. Nursing care is one of the most obvious categories, though there have been controversies (for example following the Jay report (Cmnd 7468, 1979)) about the appropriateness of nursing training to residential care.

A high level of functional specialization can, certainly, be problematic. There is little in the training of housing officers to prepare them for the kinds of demands made on them by people discharged from psychiatric institutions, and the Institute of Housing which is currently reforming the syllabus for its professional qualification, proposes to remove what little reference there is to the problems. There is no obvious reason why a doctor or nurse should know how to cope when a roof leaks. (The example is not trivial: the Normansfield report describes how the nurses moved the patients' beds and put down buckets to catch the water. Effect administration had been paralysed by poisonous relationships within the hospital. (Cmnd 7357, 1978)) The advantage of the separation of 'accommodation' and 'support' in this context is that it defines distinct roles, and the Wagner report's solution, which is a good one, is the use of a multidisciplinary team, in which functional specialisms are allied to role differentiation. This is very desirable, and it should increase the range of service, but it is not equivalent to making a residential team a completely flexible, multipurpose team. On the contrary, role differentiation works by ensuring that defined functions are carried out appropriately once common objectives have been established.

'Accommodation' and 'support' in practice come bundled together, whether we like it or not. This does not mean that the arrangements have to be completely inflexible, but there are obvious limits. It follows from the pattern of building, organization, and staffing that the scope for adaptation must be limited. Kelly holds up one residential community, for autistic people, as an example of the sort of flexibility which the Wagner report calls for: it seems to me the exception that proves the rule.

The ability to adapt and evolve in response to the changing needs of individual residents has been another aspect of the service. Thus, as the

residents have become young adults the most appropriate way of orga-
nizing care to meet individual needs has also had to change. *Somerset
Court has been extensively rebuilt in the last few years* (Kelly, 1990,
iv: my emphasis)

Clearly, it is desirable that institutions should be planned as far as
possible to take into account the developing needs of their population. But can it be realistic to commit institutions routinely to a
programme of major physical alterations? Even if the institution
can be adapted, one has to wonder whether the process of adaptation might not generate as many problems as it solves.

It is debatable too, whether this level of responsiveness is the
best way to respond to needs. Institutions are commonly established in response to a level of need in the community which
exceeds the ability of the local services to cope, and changing the
nature of the institution is likely to change the type of response
the services are able to make. One might, for example, re-equip a
home for mentally handicapped people to deal with the needs of a
group which is more profoundly handicapped, but it will not then
satisfy the needs of the client group for whom the home was first
designed. Equally, it is fairly common in half way houses for psychiatric patients to find that the residents do not wish to move on.
Unfortunately, this means that once the places have been filled,
they become unavailable to others who need short- or mid-term
placements. The whole idea of 'half way houses' is that people
should move on from them. Taken too literally, the idea of tailor-
ing services to residents' individual needs would be self-contradic-
tory; if the residents did not on the whole need the type of care
offered within the unit, they should not have been placed there.

Many of the problems stem, not from the intrinsic deficiencies
of residential care, but the inadequacy of the range and levels of
provision. Referrals are identified, and allocations made, according
to the type of service provided. The allocation of accommodation
is therefore also an allocation of particular kinds of other
resources. But there are varied reasons why a person may be
referred for care; for example, the person may simply want better
accommodation. One of the commonplaces of application to
sheltered housing is not that elderly people apply at the point
when they need support, but that they apply because the accommodation is desirable. People may want accommodation in a particular location—a factor which has been important in the provision of special accommodation for elderly people. Another possibility is that the person may need another form of support, but the
ideal for that person is not available. Availability at any particular
time depends on vacancies, and vacancies occur most frequently
where there is least demand. Services are often chosen because

they are available, even though they may be inappropriate to an individual's needs-if not wholly inappropriate, then perhaps second or third best. The argument seems to imply that more residential units are needed, of different kinds—not that residential places should not be established in the first place.

Should accommodation and support be distinct?

The case Wagner makes out for this distinction is founded in some very sound principles—in particular, the desire to undermine artificial distinctions between different kinds of care, and to introduce an element of responsiveness to need in otherwise inflexible institutions. But there are potentially negative aspects in the way the committee attempted to do this. From the point of view of residential care, the position seems well-intentioned if difficult to put into practice. From the point of view of social housing, the approach is much more destructive; it is liable to marginalize the importance of housing provision in community care. The distinction between accommodation and support legitimates a fairly widespread view that housing and accommodation can be considered quite separately from other supportive mechanisms.

Accommodation is a form of support, and often a crucial one. In the first place, accommodation is a significant need in itself. Many of the clients of special housing are, in one sense or another, especially vulnerable in that they are liable in a competitive market to find themselves in inferior housing on unfavourable terms.

Second, accommodation provides a secure basis for the development of social relationships. Physically disabled people need not only internal mobility, but access to communal facilities. For mentally handicapped people, one of the primary considerations is support for families, in which location can play a significant part. People recovering from mental illness may be at risk of a relapse, particularly if the mental illness is social in origin, a reaction to stress or isolation. In each case, the provision of adequate and appropriate accommodation is likely to be a major part of any care plan.

Third, accommodation is often an essential precondition for the delivery of other care services. This may be true simply because the accommodation is the setting in which care is in practice delivered, but it is equally important within 'community care', where the development of a treatment plan and maintenance of support within the community often depend crucially on the availability and location of accommodation. This may reflect social needs, but equally it may be true because people are unable to receive appropriate physical care if they do not have appropriately situated accommodation. In the case of discharged psychiatric patients, the maintenance of a care plan often depends on the delivery of medication either at home, or at a location near to the home: a patient who does not receive medication is liable to suffer, not simply a psychiatric breakdown, but at the same time a breakdown of social relationships. One of the most obvious failures of community care has been the incidence of homelessness among psychiatric patients—to the extent that the whole concept has been described as a cruel joke.

The dangers of attempting to separate accommodation from support can be seen in the Griffiths report on community care which came out at very nearly the same time as the Wagner report. Griffiths (1988) argued that:

> The responsibility of public housing authorities should be limited to arranging and sometimes financing and managing the 'bricks and mortar' of housing needed for community care purposes.

The report proposes a major shift in responsibility towards SSDs. At one level, this is unexceptionable: the bane of provision for community care has been the lack of adequately defined lines of accountability, and the absence, with a few notable exceptions, of clearly designated funding by which priorities could be established and initiatives undertaken. However, part of the package Griffiths offered was a shift, not only in responsibility for planning and coordination, but also the functional operations of professionals in different services. Social services would be responsible for human contact, housing for 'bricks and mortar'. This is, I think, based in a major misunderstanding on the role of housing services; it underestimates the significance of housing in people's lives, the importance of housing as a basis for provision of all kinds, and the role played by housing officers as part of the multidisciplinary team. Griffiths later retracted, stating that the important issue was to provide an appropriate administrative framework. Sadly, there is little suggestion of this in the Government's white paper, which seems if anything to be moving away from models of coordination and liaison, and scarcely considers the contribution of housing at all.

A range of options?

There are important defects in the distinction of 'accommodation' from 'support'. At the simplest level, accommodation is a form of support. This depends not simply on the physical structure of the accommodation, but on its location, its environment, and its impact on the social relationships of its residents. It is scarcely possible to separate these elements from the provision of care. At the same time, the provision of support often depends on the type of accommodation provided, and the organization, staffing, and funding associated with the particular model of care which is being offered.

There has to be some doubt as to whether the provision of supported accommodation can be seen as equivalent to 'community care'. If the support is tied to particular accommodation, and people have to move into this accommodation in order to receive the support, then the care is residential —and it seems to me on appropriate to refer to sheltered housing as a form of residential care on that basis. This does not mean that residential care does not, or should not, share some of the objectives of community care—among them 'normalization', and the fostering of independence to the greatest degree possible. But what is clear is that residential care does not rely on the same methods to achieve these aims, and that the 'care' on offer is of a different kind.

The question then remains whether it is possible to view residential care as a part of a range of options which might be drawn on as part of a package of care. On the face of it, it may still be possible—residential care provides a series of options which are not effectively open otherwise. But it is difficult, for a number of reasons, to see this as part of a 'package' of options. Residential care is itself a package, and although it may be possible to combine this type of package with others, the issues of staffing, finance, administration, and the level of needs being deal with, particularly at the more intensive levels, may make it difficult to combine this type of package effectively with other, community-based packages.

I have to express some doubts as to the success of attempts to develop an adequate range of services. Much of this scepticism is based on fairly loose impressions, conversations with professionals, discussions with service planners, and so forth, because the basic research which might establish the extent of the problems has not been done. The difficulties have been as follows. First, there seems to be a mismatch of services to needs. This follows, in part, from the historical development of residential services, and in part from the problems I have referred to in the process of referral and allocation. Equally, services are likely to become 'silted up' with clients whose needs have changed since allocation, but for whom adequate alternatives do not exist. Initially, for example, group homes were intended to act as a transitional stage for residents. In practice it can be difficult to settle a new person in with existing residents, and the homes have become permanent (Ritchie and Keegan, 1983). Half way houses seem to be developing the same way.

Second, part of the implication of the concept of a range of services is that services have to over-respond to needs. If there is no spare capacity, the options do not exist for new cases. But there is underprovision in many places—for example, for discharged psychiatric patients and, if excess demand is a sign, for frail elderly people. Where overprovision does exist, as it may in child care, prevention is usually dealt with fairly ruthlessly by cutting resources—unless, of course, the overprovision is in the private sector, where it can be tolerated as long as the accommodation produces an economic rate of return.

Third, there are difficulties in establishing appropriate professional coordination. The Wagner proposals depend, like much of community care, on the operation of multidisciplinary teams, and coordination and liaison. But the idea of developing a new range or pattern of services ignores the existing framework, which has services and institutions in place, and is administered by people with particular approaches and skills.

The modification of these schemes to expand the range of options is an ideal, but what is not clear is how to move from the present situation to the desired one. There is also the question of whether it might be better—in the sense both of more acceptable and more practical to move to second-best alternatives. These might include more centralized resources, different uses of existing residential facilities, or even an expansion and upgrading of residential care rather than aiming, as seems to happen now, for the best and ending up with services which are third rate or worse.

An agenda for research

The existing literature on options for community seems to me to overlook many of these issues. The consideration of the cost-effectiveness of the 'balance of care' in varying kinds of provision seems promising (eg Audit Inspectorate, 1983, 1986; Challis and Davies 1986), and the Audit Inspectorate's 1983 consideration of mental handicap is one of the best examples of attempting to consider services as a whole. One might think that the establishment of which options are cost-effective for each individual would lead to the appropriate matching of individuals to services. But the issues of process have not been adequately addressed, and it is difficult to see how the ideal allocation of people to services can ever be achieved.

It seems appropriate, in view of the yawning gaps in the available information, to conclude with an agenda for research. The review of literature on residential care in the Wagner report is enormously helpful, and there is little point in duplicating it here, but it is mainly concerned with two principal areas—the operation of residential care itself, and the operation of residential care in relation to the needs of particular groups. Care plans have to be constructed from a range of options available from various kinds of services and sources of provision. In arguing that residential care has to be seen as a range of options to be used flexibly in the same way as different kinds of community care provision, the Wagner report breaks new ground. But much of the empirical material to establish how this range of options might work in practice as a range, rather than a focus on the success or failure of constituent elements, does not as yet exist.

The first stage is to seek to investigate the situation as it develops, to establish what the processes are through which the range of options is being developed, and what problems might be arising. There are several problems in developing research at this level. Much of the provision and funding for research are based on the small scale. The consumers who tend to be featured in such research are often those who are tied to the system, and not those who are outside its scope. A focus on aggregated individual results confuses consumer preference with social priorities: I suspect the result has been to overestimate the need for certain kinds of residential care, like sheltered housing, but that has to be established. It disaggregates results which should be considered collectively; the small scale of much work has led to a blinkered approach in which certain options, like centralized peripatetic resources, or even significant improvements in residential provisions, are foreclosed. Lastly, it presupposes that services are actually going to respond at the individual level, when much of what I have written suggests that this is not the way in which services are actually going to be delivered or organized.

Equally, there are problems in focusing on the provision of existing services, because existing services are fragmented and still relatively uncoordinated. An emphasis on services can help to show what services are supposed to do, and what role they are actually playing, but there is little potential in analysis of particular services to identify how effectively they are dealing with the range of needs. The kind of research I am arguing for would focus on administrative issues, at the level of social planning.

The next stage of a research protocol would be to consider some possible responses to the kinds of problems outlined in this paper. The problem is not so much to outline the formation of an alternative ideal model; ideal models abound. The problems which need to be resolved are mainly those of process rather than principle—how to get from where we are to any position which seems more desirable. At this stage of knowledge, I have very little idea what the solutions might be.

References

Anderson D 1981 Community care: why are people so reluctant to bring it to life? *Mind Out*, Sept: 18–21

Audit Inspectorate 1983 *Community care: care of mentally handicapped people* HMSO, London

Audit Inspectorate 1986 *Making a reality of community care.* HMSO, London

Bayley M 1973 *Mental Handicap and Community Care,* Routledge, Kegan Paul, London

Clapham D, Smith S J 1990 Housing policy and 'special needs' *Policy and Politics* **18**: 193–206

Cmnd 7357 1978 *Report of the committee of inquiry into Normansfield hospital.* HMSO, London

Cmnd 7468 1979 *Report of the committee of inquiry into mental handicap nursing and care.* HMSO, London

Challis D, Davies B 1986 *Matching resources to needs in community care.* Gower, Aldershot

Griffiths R 1988 *Community care: agenda for action.* HMSO,1989 London,Cm 849 *Caring for people: community care in the next decade and beyond.* HMSO, London

Kelly D 1990 Practising Wagner. *Community Care* 1st February: iii-iv

Martin J P 1984 *Hospitals in Trouble.* Blackwell, Oxford

Meteyard B 1985 When a home is not a home, *Community Care,* 24th Oct

Ritchie J, Keegan J 1983 *Housing for mentally ill and mentally handicapped people.* Department of the Environment, London

Spicker P 1989 *Social housing and the social services* Longman, London

Wagner G 1988 *Residential care: a positive choice.* HMSO, London

9 Housing and community care

David Clapham

Introduction

For large numbers of people with chronic health problems the policy prescription is 'community care'. Therefore, many people with physical disabilities or learning difficulties; those suffering from some form of mental illness; and those who are considered to be vulnerable because of physical disabilities, or illness or the social isolation associated with old age now find themselves 'in the community' rather than being incarcerated in institutions. And this policy direction commands widespread, although not universal, support from politicians, academics, and pressure groups, even if there is not an equivalent agreement about what 'community care' can, or should entail in practice. The term 'community care' has become almost meaningless because it can cover such a wide variety of different objectives, priorities and policies. For example, what balance should there be between care by statutory services and care by family or neighbors? To what extent should people live in supported accommodation as against living in 'ordinary' housing?

The most fundamental issues are largely sidestepped in Government pronouncements on community care. In the white paper *Caring for People* (Cmnd 849, 1989) (p 3) community care is defined as follows:

> Community care means providing the services and support which people who are affected by problems of ageing, mental illness, mental handicap, or physical or sensory disability need to be able to live as independently as possible in their own homes, or in 'homely' settings in the community.

The emphasis on 'homes' and 'homely settings' shows the importance attached to housing in community care.

If dependent people are to be helped to continue living in the community, then their homes must be places where it is possible to provide the care they need. The government believes that housing is a vital component of community care and it is often the key to independent living. (Cmnd 849, 1989 p 25)

In addition, it is stipulated in the white paper that SSDs must collaborate with housing agencies in drawing up the new mandatory community care plans.

The importance explicitly attached to housing is a step forward when compared with previous Government pronouncements but it is not reflected in the space devoted to housing issues in the white paper, which is less than a single page in a document of over 100 pages. Here, discussion of the role of housing in community care is short and superficial. Similarly, in the Griffiths report, to which the white paper is a response, discussion of housing issues is given three paragraphs, and these are focused on the proposed restriction of the role of housing organizations to the provision of 'bricks and mortar'. Likewise, in *Making a Reality of Community Care* (Audit Commission, 1986) housing is mentioned only as a service which needs to be integrated with health and personal social services. There is no discussion of what kind of housing policy or housing services are appropriate for community care.

The aim of this chapter is to examine the implicit assumptions about the role of housing made in the previously mentioned reports on community care and in Government community care policies. It is argued that the approach taken is an unduly narrow one which focuses on a few marginal housing policies and forms of provision at the expense of 'mainstream' policies and programmes. The limitations of this restricted approach are outlined and an alternative focus is put forward which places the objectives of community care at the centre of housing policy. Some 'mainstream' policies and programmes which have implications for community care and which form an agenda for research and policy are then briefly examined.

The Government's agenda

In the white paper *Caring for People*, the Government focuses on three different areas where housing has a contribution to make towards community care.

First, there is mention of Government support for the provision by local authorities and housing associations of 'staying put' and 'care and repair' schemes for older owner occupiers which provide advice to older people on how to keep their homes in good repair, and on how to finance repairs and adaptations by, for example, using the capital tied up in their property (Wheeler, 1985). Mention is also made in the white paper of the powers in the *Local Government and Housing Act* which enables local housing authorities to provide assistance to enable older people, or those caring for them, to undertake minor works in their homes.

Secondly, attention is drawn to grants which are available to help disabled people carry out structural adaptations to their homes and to provisions in the *Local Government and Housing Act,* for an income related disabled facilities grant. Local authorities will give mandatory grants where improvements are needed to give access to basic amenities in and around the home. Discretionary grants can be made to make dwellings suitable for a disabled person.

Finally, there is mention of special provision for severely disabled or older disabled people. The particular forms mentioned are wheelchair housing, core and cluster developments, and sheltered and very sheltered housing. Presumably these kinds of provision are what is meant in the white paper by 'homely settings' in the community.

All of these programmes share a number of characteristics. First, they have relatively small amounts of resources devoted to them. Second, they are specifically targeted on groups such as older people or mentally handicapped people. Third, they are directed towards the needs which are implicitly held to be distinctive to one or more of these groups. And finally, they are secondary to the main housing policies and programmes pursued by the Government, such as the continued support for owner-occupation and the restructuring of public rented housing. In short, these are 'special' policies designed to ease some of the immediate problems of people who are included in categories such as 'mentally handicapped' or 'physically disabled'.

Using 'special' policies simultaneously to target and ration public resources has some advantages to the people who benefit from them, but can also have many disadvantages (Clapham and Smith, 1990). The targeting or rationing of resources on the basis of group identity can lead to the provision of services which directly meet some needs of some people. An example of this may be sheltered housing for older people which provides a mix of housing and support services which can meet effectively many needs of some older people who have physical disabilities or who are isolated and vulnerable to emergency situations (Clapham and Munro, 1990). This form of provision is popular with most of the older people who use it and there is substantial demand for places in sheltered housing schemes in both the public and private sectors. Nevertheless, only a small minority of older people benefit from this form of provision and even for those who do there is a price to pay.

The desire to target resources means that there have to be rules of inclusion and exclusion. In other words, there have to be definitions of old age or physical disability, which delineate the boundaries between those who benefit from the special policies and programmes and those who do not. These standard definitions by their very nature are bound to be arbitrary and inflexible. For example, old age is usually defined as starting at the state defined retirement age, even though the physical processes of ageing vary considerably in their impact on different people. Two people aged 65 may have very different problems and abilities, and a 60 year old may, on occasion, be more frail and dependent than a 70 year old.

Targeting is considered necessary to make the most of the resources available and to separate 'deserving' groups from the 'undeserving'. However, even if a person is lucky enough to be categorized within a 'deserving' group, membership carries with it the implicit assumption that they share a set of special problems and needs with other members of the group. In other words, to be categorized as 'old' means the implicit acceptance of all the images which are associated with the category. The group as a whole has to justify its preferential status by drawing attention to the enormity and urgency of the needs of its members. This leads to the reinforcement of negative stereotyping and to stigmatisation. Older people are characterized as problems in need of special assistance rather than integral members of society. Their categorization and perceived special needs for special policies and forms of provision mean that they are separated out from other members of society by the way in which they are treated. Some older people do have problems which require different forms or degrees of help, but often these problems are shared with people in other age groups. For example, physical disabilities or low income are characteristics shared by many younger people.

The categorization of older people leads to a view that it is old age which is 'the problem' rather than low income or physical disability which may accompany old age for some people, but which many other people may experience. The identification of old age as the decisive causal factor in the need for special services has the effect of limiting eligibility to deserving groups and diverting attention away from the functioning of the housing system. In other words it is old age which is perceived as the cause of housing problems not the inability of the housing system to provide decent housing for those on low incomes. This focus allows state aid to be provided in ways which do not alter the fundamental characteristics of the housing system. This is an important point because as the concern about community care has grown and the number of 'special' housing policies and programmes has increased, changes have been made to the housing system which have led to increased difficulties for people in need of community care—a point which will be expanded in the next section.

In summary, the current Government's approach to housing and community care is through the adoption of special policies and programmes designed for, and restricted to, these groups. The major criticisms of this approach are that it can lead to stigmatization by reinforcing negative stereotypes associated with these groups; that, by its discrimination, it tends to set apart the groups from other housing consumers (in some forms of policy such as the provision of special forms of accommodation, this separation may also be physical), and finally that it diverts attention away from other more important factors operating in the housing system as a whole, which have major implications for community care.

These factors are important given the stated emphasis in community care of people living as independently as possible and enabling them to achieve their full potential. Therefore, the Government's current approach to the housing needs of community care groups has effects which contradict the stated aims of community care policy.

Towards an alternative approach

Community care, in the words of the Government, is concerned with keeping people in their own homes, fostering their independence, and enabling them to fulfil their potential. Crucially, it is also concerned with integration into society rather than exclusion from it—an aim which is implicit in government statements about independence and potential, but not made explicit. It is implicit because it is not possible for a person to be independent and to fulfil their potential if they are excluded from mainstream society. Exclusion brings with it stigma and a low valuation of a person's worth in society which can only serve to influence the opportunities which a person has. These concerns were brought to the forefront in the concept of normalization. Tyne identified its aims as:

> first helping handicapped people to gain skills and characteristics, and to experience a lifestyle, which is valued in our society and to have opportunities for using skills and expressing individuality in choice; secondly, regardless of people's handicaps, providing services in settings and in ways which are valued in our society and supporting people to participate genuinely in the mainstream of life. (Tyne, 1982, p 151)

138

Although usually applied to policy towards people with learning difficulties, normalization is a useful guide to community care policy in general. It shows clearly that policies and programmes have to be provided in a way which seeks to minimize differences in the treatment of older people from that given to others. Targeting in the form of special policies directed at 'deserving' groups provides support in a way which is based on the assumption that different treatment is appropriate between different categories of people while the same kinds of treatment is required by each individual within a given category. For those singled out for 'special' treatment, therefore, the resultant benefits are offset by the stigmatization and separation from mainstream society which follow from it.

The logical consequence of this is that the policy emphasis should be switched away from 'special' policies to an examination of 'mainstream' or universal policies and policy instruments in order to examine their potential for contributing towards the aims of community care. In other words, the objectives of community care should become key housing objectives and constitute criteria by which the performance of the housing system as a whole is judged.

A comprehensive examination of the housing system is beyond the scope of this chapter. However, in the next few sections some areas of policy will be outlined which would seem to offer opportunities for mainstream housing initiatives to make a contribution towards the objectives of community care. They are also areas where current policy or practice works against these objectives and serves to mitigate if not completely offset the impact of special needs policies.

Distribution of housing subsidy

People in need of community care usually have very low incomes, because their problems are likely to make it difficult or impossible to take up employment. Those who are in employment may find difficulty in competing for jobs at times of high unemployment (which have characterized the 1980s) and even if successful may be restricted to relatively low paid jobs. The same general picture applies to people living in a household with a carer. There is substantial evidence that caring by a family member, usually a woman, can lead to the carer not being able to take up employment, or being restricted in the type of job they can take. This may result in a low income (Parker, 1990).

It must be stressed that this is only a general picture. People in need of community care can be in very different financial circumstances. For example, some older people may have little or no savings and be dependent on state benefits. Others may have substantial savings and investments and a high income from those investments. However, there is little systematic information on the relationship between income and housing expenditure for those receiving community care. For example, we do not know what proportion of people with a mental illness living at home receive housing benefit or mortgage interest tax relief. Without crucial knowledge of this kind it is possible only to make sweeping generalizations about the impact of the housing finance system on those in need of community care. However, in general, any housing policy which discriminates against people with low incomes is likely to have an adverse impact on many of the most vulnerable people in need of community care. Therefore, a regressive housing subsidy policy will generally run counter to the objectives of community care and a progressive housing subsidy policy will help the achievement of those objectives.

Much has been written about the amount and incidence of housing subsidies and no consensus exists on the details. However, there is little dispute about the general picture. In the 1980s general subsidies to council housing have been almost completely phased out and the process of cutting those payable to housing associations has begun (Malpass, 1990). The major subsidy to those living in rented housing, where those on low incomes are concentrated, is housing benefit which has seen repeated cuts in real terms in the late 1980s (Clapham et al, 1990).

The amount of money made available in housing benefit is small when compared with the tax relief given to owner-occupiers. Estimates put tax relief on mortgage interest payments at £5.5 billion in 1988–89 (Building Societies Association, 1989) compared to the £3.66 billion spent on housing benefit (Hills, 1989). In comparison, according to the white paper £4.5 million was spent in 1987–88 on grants to enable disabled people to carry out structural adaptations to their housing.

Therefore, the targeting of resources towards community care groups highlighted in the white paper has been associated with a general subsidy climate which is not helpful to community care objectives. Much Government help which could be used to aid those on low incomes is channelled towards owner-occupiers with those on the highest incomes and the largest mortgages (up to the limit of £30,000) receiving most help. Further, the resources devoted to special community care schemes are a very small proportion of the overall total. Without systematic information on the housing costs and subsidies of those receiving community care, it is not possible to make a detailed criticism of the existing system and propose solutions to deal with particular problems. However, the lack of information is in itself a good indication of the little interest shown in this important area.

Tenure choice

Over the last ten years there has been a concerted effort by the Government to change the tenure structure of the British housing system by expanding the owner-occupied sector (and to a lesser extent the private rented sector) and reducing the size of the public rented sector. Whereas policies designed to reinvigorate the private rented sector have not succeeded in reversing the longstanding decline in this tenure (it has declined from 10 per cent of households in 1979 to 6 per cent in 1987), those directed at the owner-occupied sector have led to a growth from 53 per cent of households in 1978 to 63 per cent in 1987, according to figures from the *General Household Survey*. The expansion of owner-occupation has been partly achieved through the shrinkage of the public rented sector from 34 per cent of households in 1979 to 26 per cent in 1987.

These changes in the tenure structure are a deliberate result of Government policies which have adopted a carrot and stick approach to enable and encourage households to enter owner-occupation and to encourage existing and potential council tenants to spurn the sector. Incentives to enter owner-occupation have included the right-to-buy given to most council and housing association tenants (Forrest and Murie, 1988). Those who have been in the sector for more than three years can take advantage of generous discounts to buy their house. There are also other schemes such as transferable discounts (where tenants can purchase another dwelling) and rent into mortgage schemes (where tenants' rent payments are transformed into payments to 'buy off' a proportion of the equity). Local councils have also been encouraged to sell their properties to private developers usually for rehabilitation and resale into owner-occupation. In addition, measures have been taken to increase the supply of owner-occupied housing by removing some restrictions in the planning process and on building standards (Booth and Crook, 1986). Housing associations have been encouraged to build or rehabilitate properties for sale and local authorities have been encouraged to help private developers.

In the public sector restrictions have been placed on capital investment which have meant that new building has been reduced to a very low level and many councils do not have enough resources to keep all their properties in good structural repair and containing modern facilities (Cantle, 1986). In addition, the Government has reduced subsidies it has paid to local authorities and has prohibited local authorities from subsiding council housing from local taxation. Action has also been taken to force up rents (Malpass, 1990). The consequences to the Exchequer in the form of increased housing benefit payments have been limited by reducing eligibility to the benefit and by forcing some local authorities to cover some of the cost from rental income.

The consequences of these policies have been an increase in the trend evident since the 1950s of a polarization between owner-occupation and council housing and the residualization of council housing (for a review of this trend see Clapham and English, 1987). Owner-occupation is the desired tenure of most people and those able to enter the tenure are doing so. Inevitably, in these circumstances council housing is viewed by most people as a second best tenure inhabited by low income households who are not able to buy their own house. The deterioration in the physical condition of the public sector stock and in the housing management service offered to tenants have reinforced this second-best image.

Tenure change has a number of consequences for community care, both for those who attain the goal of owner occupation and for those who are forced to rely on council housing. Because many of those in need of community care are likely to be without employment, and dependent on state benefits, or in low paid jobs, their relatively modest incomes are likely to consign most of them to the public rented sector. Rising rents, the scaling down of housing benefits and deteriorating conditions in the sector are of obvious importance to community care. Also important is the increasing stigma attached to the sector. The deteriorating service, the diminishing size of the sector and the increasing concentration of low income households within the sector have reinforced the view espoused by the Government that it caters for 'social cases'. In its statements on housing policy the Government is clearly aware of the decline of council housing, which it blames on local councils, and identifies council housing with a range of social evils.

> In some areas the system has provided good quality housing and management. But in many big cities local authority housing operations are so large that they inevitably risk becoming distant and bureaucratic. Insensitive design and bad management have alienated tenants and left housing badly maintained. As the quality of the housing and of its environment has declined, so a wide range of social problems has emerged; crime and violence have increased; many people have left for better opportunities elsewhere; local enterprise and employment have disappeared; and whole communities have slipped into a permanent dependence on the welfare system from which it is extremely difficult for people to escape. (DoE, 1987)

The problem is that the provision of housing to meet the needs of community care groups, whether in the form of 'special provision' or of 'ordinary' housing, is most likely to be made in the public sector. For example, the only form of special provision in the private sector which is reasonably common is sheltered housing for older people. Even in this case provision is small (if growing rapidly) when compared to the public sector. Of course, many older people and other community care groups are able to attain owner-occupation (of which more later) but because of low incomes they are likely to be overrepresented in the public sector. For example, most patients discharged from institutions for the mentally ill or mentally handicapped are likely to gain their first experience of 'the community' in public rented housing either in a hostel or similar 'special scheme' run by the public or voluntary sector; or in a mainstream tenancy in the public or voluntary sector. Access to owner-occupation will be difficult, unless they are able to build up the savings and income necessary to purchase a house, as well as the skills and knowledge required to run and maintain it. For the vast majority who will not be able to enter owner-occupation, if being part of the public sector is likely to condemn them to living in poor housing conditions, in a deprived and deteriorating neighbourhood, subject to a poor service from the landlord, and stigmatized by and cut off spatially and socially from people in other tenures—then the objectives of normalization and community care are unlikely to be met.

Life may not be rosy either for those who attain the goal of owner-occupation. The myths surrounding this tenure tend to obscure the fact that not all parts of the sector enjoy the good housing conditions and wealth accumulation with which owner-occupation is associated in the public mind (Forrest, et al 1990). Because of their low income many people subject to community care find themselves in this part of the sector where they may be trapped in deteriorating physical conditions without access to resources to deal with the situation.

Even those who are able to enter better parts of the private sector may find that owner-occupation creates difficulties for them. For example, any disruption in income can have serious consequences for someone paying a mortgage. Temporary support is available to meet interest payments, but if the situation continues, action can be taken to repossess a house and homelessness can ensue. Even for people who own their house outright, a reduction in income due, for example, to retirement can lead to problems in having enough income to keep the property in good repair. There have been responses from public, private and voluntary agencies to help deal with such problems. For example, care and repair schemes can provide advice to older people and enable them to apply for improvement grants and to convert some of the wealth stored in their houses into income through a secured loan. However, solutions such as this are only available to a few older people and would need to be expanded considerably in scope to make them available to all older people in a way that enables them to gain such help.

The push towards owner-occupation means that more and more people in need of community care will be owner-occupiers—a status which may not necessarily be a suitable one for them in its present form. Some measures can be taken to alleviate problems by, for example, protecting people from repossession of their homes or by making benefits available to cover repayment of the capital as well as the interest. However, the only real answer is to adopt a tenure policy which accepts that some people will be more suited to renting and would choose this option if this sector were not stigmatized and had good quality dwellings available which were well managed and maintained.

Reform of the housing association movement

Because of financial restrictions, there have been substantial reductions in the capacity of local councils to build new rented housing and to convert their existing stock. Therefore, attention has increasingly turned towards housing associations as a means of providing rented housing in general and accommodation for those in need of community care in particular. Housing associations, often in collaboration with statutory or voluntary social service agencies, have been in the forefront of the development of innovative forms of provision for community care groups. They have been able to do this because of support and generous subsidies from the Government. However, in 1989 the Government, whilst still expressing strong support for the sector, changed the financial regime for housing associations (Kearns, 1988). The changes were designed to lower the rates of subsidy paid by the Government and to encourage associations to seek loans from private sector institutions to support their activities. Also, rents are to rise from 'fair rents' to 'affordable rents', although it has proved difficult to define what this will mean in practice. The new financial system is intended to be flexible, so that levels of subsidy and rents will vary between individual schemes. This makes it even more difficult than usual to foresee the impact the changes will have. Nevertheless, it is clear that there is nothing in the changes which will make it easier for associations to provide community care and further, there are some aspects which give rise to concern.

According to the Government the new system of private sector loans and reduced subsidy will not apply to all schemes. The impression has been given that 'special needs' schemes, such as hostels for mentally handicapped people, will still be given the same level of grant as previously. However, it is not clear how widely this exemption will be drawn. For example, will all sheltered housing schemes for older people still attract the previously high rates of subsidy? It would be easy in this case for the Government to argue that at least some schemes could be aimed at older people with higher incomes who could pay higher 'affordable rents', and so the subsidy element could be reduced and an element of private loan introduced.

Also, although some schemes are still to be given the traditionally high levels of subsidy, the Government's stated objective is that the average level of grant should fall substantially from its present level—although there is considerable confusion over the level which is desirable and whether it is feasible. It is not clear at what level this averaging process will operate. Does it mean that a housing association specializing in schemes for mentally ill people will also have to produce some 'mainstream' schemes with private finance to keep their average rate of grant down, or will the averaging only take place at a higher level (national or regional)? If the latter, will the need to reduce average levels mean that there will be pressure to reduce the number of high-granted special schemes? What impact will the need to reduce grant levels have on mixed schemes which are predominantly mainstream but involve some special needs provision?

Finally, the Government through its new financial regime has shifted the risk arising from unforeseen circumstances away from itself and onto the associations. In other words, if there are cost overruns on building work, they are borne by the association and not, as previously, met through grant. More importantly, for this discussion, the same principle applies for revenue costs. Thus, if rent arrears levels or vacancy rates are higher than expected, the shortfall in rental income has to be met by the association. This could make associations more 'risk averse' than they have been in the past and make them more reluctant to offer tenancies to potentially problematic tenants amongst whose number could be people in need of community care.

It is clear that the need for housing associations to make an effective contribution to community care was not at the forefront of the minds of those planning the changes to housing associations. Other objectives such as the desire to make government subsidy stretch further, increasing rents and encouraging associations to compete with local authorities were the key considerations. The result has been changes which will not make it easier for housing associations to meet community care needs and could result in their task being made more difficult.

When these changes are coupled with the parlous state of much council housing and the stubborn resistance of private landlordism to expand in the way the Government wishes, it becomes apparent that rented accommodation in any form is becoming more difficult to find and a less desirable option for households. This means that many people in need of community care are finding it more difficult to find appropriate rented accommodation and some are reduced to homelessness and even sleeping rough. Even those who manage to obtain rented accommodation can be faced with poor standards. Consequently, more and more of those who can barely afford it are being forced to look towards owner-occupation with the dangers which this can have for vulnerable people.

Housing management

The appropriate methods of managing rented housing have been debated for at least 150 years (Clapham, et al 1990). For example, as far back as the 1840s Octavia Hill criticized the management practices of private landlords and model dwelling companies and put forward and practised a coherent alternative to their methods which emphasized the importance of dealing with tenants as individuals rather than concentrating entirely on property management. Octavia Hill's approach was for managers to build up a personal relationship with tenants and to use this to encourage them to conform to her moral code as well as to look after the property. Housing management was seen as a form of social work and indeed Hill was a member of the Charity Organization Society which was one of the forerunners of modern social work. Hill's method was influential at the time amongst model dwelling companies, but with the introduction of council housing on a large scale in the interwar years, local councils commonly rejected her methods in favour of the creation of standardized administrative procedures designed to look after the property and to treat people in an impersonal, uniform and equitable way. Thus, the social work focus on people as individuals was largely rejected and the two professions adopted very different *modus operandi*.

Debates about the appropriate focus of housing management have continued and the role of housing managers has changed at different times. In particular, concern about a more socially orientated focus has repeatedly emerged, usually at times when the role of the public sector has been to house the poorest members of society. The current residualization of public housing outlined earlier has led to just such a debate, and there have been some changes in housing management practice designed to cope with the pressures with which public landlords now find themselves confronted. Despite this debate and activity, the nature of housing management remains in essence what it has been since the beginning of council housing. This inertia and reluctance to change is worrying because it means that public landlords are ill-equipped to deal with the challenges which community poses for them.

For example, the prevailing wisdom in housing management is for allocation policies to based on the idea of 'allocation according to need'. This is a meaningless phrase which is difficult to put into practice (Clapham and Kintrea, 1987). Nevertheless it has come to be associated with allocation systems based on the award of points for particular household characteristics or features of their housing and other circumstances. Such systems are designed to reduce discretion to a minimum and to ensure that each case is dealt with in an impersonal, uniform and equitable way.

In practice, such systems are inflexible and are unable to take into account the complexities of the needs, desires and circumstances of individual households. Such systems tend to result in substantial segregation within the public stock (Clapham and Kintrea, 1986). In other words, households in similar circumstances and with similar attributes are likely to find themselves housed together in particular neighbourhoods. For example, older households are likely to be heavily concentrated in particular parts of the public sector stock. Their children will almost certainly have had to move away to other areas to get their own houses.

One tenant management cooperative in Glasgow found that 80 per cent of its members were over retirement age as a consequence of the citywide allocation policy. Therefore, the cooperative introduced its own local policy which, although still based largely on housing need, gives some priority to relatives of existing tenants. They justify this on the basis that they are recreating a close community which was destroyed by housing management practices. They aim to enable families to live in close proximity so that children can more easily provide support for their elderly parents when needed and parents with young children can call on their relatives to help. In other words, they were keen to rekindle the family and community ties which can make care by the community possible.

This example shows the impact which housing management practices can have on community care, but there is considerable resistance amongst the housing profession to change. Initiatives such as the local lettings policy outlined above are commonly criticized as being unfair and elitist. Nevertheless, housing managers are being forced to change their methods of working as they are confronted with the problems posed by their tenants who are increasingly made up of people in need of community care. Griffiths in his report to the Government on community care stated that housing agencies should be solely concerned with 'bricks and mortar' and that the responsibility for community care lay with social services agencies. However, such a clear cut separation of responsibilities is not possible because of the interlinked nature of housing and other needs. It is in the interests of housing agencies to ensure that the care needs of their tenants are met because they have to bear many of the consequences of them not being met. For example, if a person suffering from a mental illness does not receive appropriate support they may not be able to keep their house in a reasonable condition, or they may cause problems with neighbours, or they may not be able to manage their finances appropriately and thereby get in arrears with their rental payments. All of these are problems with which housing managers will have to deal.

It is, however, unlikely that housing managers will be able to cope with the multifaceted requirements of people in need of community care. Many other skills may be required which are better provided by social workers, home helps, nurses, and other domiciliary support staff. Nonetheless, it is important that housing managers have a knowledge and understanding of what others can contribute, and that there are effective means of communication and coordination between the different professions or occupations. Relations between social workers and housing managers are generally poor. There is a mutual distrust, suspicion and even antagonism based on fundamentally different professional values and working practices. The divide may narrow if housing managers change their methods of working in response to the demands of community care. The new role of 'case management' to be given to SSDs may also change the nature of the relationship and improve communication and coordination. Nevertheless, there is a substantial gulf to be bridged if community care is to be provided in an effective and coherent way and housing managers are to play their full part in this.

The recognition of the important role that housing management could play in community care was one factor behind the widespread rejection by housing professionals and commentators of the Griffiths suggestion for the division of responsibilities. However, there have been few positive steps towards recasting the role and practice of housing management in order to make the valuable contribution to community care which is possible. The changes needed are far reaching and involve organizational structures, housing management procedures and, perhaps most importantly, the skills and knowledge of housing managers. At present the training offered to housing managers does not reflect the demands which community care places on them, and so most housing managers are ill equipped for the role they are being increasingly forced to accept.

Conclusion

In the white paper *Caring for People* the Government has taken a major step forward by declaring the importance of housing in meeting the objectives of community care. However, the impact of this declaration is lost because of the lack of space devoted to housing issues and the narrow view taken of the range of housing policies and programmes which have an impact on community care.

Through its choice of housing issues highlighted in the white paper, it is clear that the Government views the achievement of community care objectives as requiring merely some fairly small additions to existing housing policy which are targeted exclusively on those needing community care. Such an approach has many drawbacks. It requires people to be categorized into groups and leaves them open to the unthinking acceptance by others of group characteristics and stereotypes which do not reflect individuals' abilities or needs and can paint an overly negative picture of their position. The approach also leads to the provision of specific policy and programmes designed to meet 'group' needs which, although of benefit to some group members, can serve to hinder the achievement of community care objectives by separating out individuals from the rest of the community in a social and often a spatial way. The discriminatory treatment offered to those in need of community care would be more acceptable if it was built onto a housing system which already successfully met most needs.

However, this is not the case and perhaps the most damning indictment of the present approach is that the beneficial impact of discriminatory policy is overwhelmed by the workings of the housing system which does not provide well for people in need of community care, many of whom are consigned to a residualized and stigmatized public sector and offered little help from a housing subsidy regime which provides most to better off owner-occupiers. There is doubt whether those in community care will be able to rely on the housing association movement in the way they have done in the recent past. And in all the rented sectors they are likely to be confronted with a housing management system which is not geared to meet their needs and to come into contact with housing managers who are ill equipped to deal with their problems.

This situation can only be rectified if the objectives of community care are seen not as relating to just a few marginal housing policies but rather as objectives which underpin the whole of housing policy. Since 1979 housing has been viewed as predominantly a marketed commodity rather than as a social service (Clapham, et al, 1990). Consequently social policy objectives have not been at the forefront of government concerns over housing. However, until community care objectives are seen to be at the heart of the Government housing policy, housing will not play the major role in community care of which it is capable of. And those in need of community care will continue to miss the support which they need to live independent and fulfilling lives.

References

Audit Commission 1986 *Making a reality of community care.* Audit Commission, London

Booth P, and Crook A Eds, 1986 *Low cost home ownership* Gower, Aldershot

Building Societies Association 1989 *Housing Finance* **No 1** Building Societies Association, London

Cantle E 1986 The Deterioration of Public Sector Housing in Malpass P Ed, *The housing crisis* Croom Helm, London

Clapham D, English J Eds, 1987 *Public housing: Current trends and future developments.* Croom Helm, London

Clapham D, Kemp P, Smith S J 1990 *Housing and social policy.* Macmillan, London

Clapham D, Kintrea K 1986 Rationing choice and constraint: the allocation of public housing in Glasgow. *Journal of Social Policy* 15 : 51–67

Clapham D, Kintrea K 1987 Housing allocation and the role of the public rented sector. *Discussion Paper* **14** Centre for Housing Research Glasgow

Clapham D, Munro M 1990 Ambiguities and contradictions in the provision of sheltered housing for older people. *Journal of Social Policy* **19** : 27–45

Clapham D, Smith S J 1990 Housing policy and 'special needs', *Policy and Politics* **18** : 193–206

Department of the Environment 1987 *Housing: the government's proposals.* HMSO, London

Forrest R, Murie A 1988 *Selling the welfare state.* Croom Helm London

Forrest R, Murie A, Williams P 1990 *Home ownership.* George Allen and Unwin, London

Griffiths R 1988 *Community care: agenda for action.* HMSO, London

Hills J 1989 Distributional effects of housing subsidies in the United Kingdom. *Discussion Paper* **44** Suntory-Toyota International Centre for Economics and Related Disciplines, London School of Economics London

Kearns A 1988 Affordable rents and flexible HAG: new finance for housing associations. *Discussion Paper* **17** Centre for Housing Research, Glasgow

Malpass P 1990 *Reshaping housing policy: subsidies, rents and residualisation.* Routledge, London

Parker G 1990 *With due care and attention.* 2nd ed Family Policy Studies Center

Tyne A 1982 Community care and mentally handicapped people. In Walker A Ed, Community Care Blackwell and Martin Robertson, Oxford

Wheeler R 1985 *Don't move we have got you covered.* Institute of Housing, London

PART III
HEALTH CARE
FOR
HOMELESS PEOPLE

10 Homeless women and pregnancy

Nigel Shanks

Introduction

Historically, the medical care of the poor and the homeless has been, at best, perfunctory and has depended largely on the efforts of sympathetic individuals. The Beveridge report (1942) on social insurance and allied services concluded that there must be the provision of health care within a broader framework of social services that would free the general populace of the 'giant evils of Want, Disease, Ignorance, Squalor and Idleness'. Nevertheless, a walk around any city at night is all that is needed to demonstrate that there is a population whose existence is not commensurate with the ideals envisaged by Beveridge, or those who today have responsibility for providing the various welfare services. Indeed, 30 years ago Sargaison (1954) identified that: 'the main defect in the welfare legislation is found in the lack of facilities for dealing with illnesses in elderly lodging house men'.

A major objective of the NHS at its inception was to provide readily accessible medical care to everyone, thus reducing inequalities in health. That objective remains. Given the substantial evidence on inequalities, however, it would be perverse to avoid the conclusion that the lowest social groups have relatively bigger health needs yet, even now, receive fewer and lower quality health services.

The idea of social class has some meaning for most people, but it is limited at the level of social policy, and is inadequate for planning health programmes. The Black report concluded that people in social class IV and V had a lower state of health than those in social class I. The report relied heavily on mortality rates because of a comparative paucity of data on morbidity, and on the use of health care related to social classes. The difference in health status was ascribed primarily to a self-perpetuating cycle of socioeco-

155

nomic deprivation. The recommendations, relating mainly to social engineering, were not endorsed by the Government because of the enormous cost.

There is increasing evidence that excess mortality may be associated with adverse socioeconomic circumstances (Carstairs and Morris 1989). This has special relevance for the homeless, especially as measures of deprivation apparently provide a powerful basis for the explanation of health differences.

The problem of medical services for inner city areas is attracting serious and increasing interest. The larger cities tend to attract vagrants and other homeless people where they are housed in hostels, lodging houses, and bed and breakfast accommodation, some of which are often in various states of decay as well as being overcrowded

This unfortunate state of affairs means that living conditions are usually poor or, frankly, bad, and are consequently inimical to the maintenance of a state of good health. These conditions accentuate the hazards of city life. Analyses of disease trends show that the environment is the primary determinant of the state of general health in any population (Winkelstein 1972). Additional factors such as poverty, housing, employment and the environment contribute more than medical care to the variance in health indices (Metcalfe 1981, Marsh and Channing 1986). Nevertheless, so wide are the social class and geographical differences documented in the Black report that any improvement in the provision of care for those most at risk should result in the saving of lives and the relief of suffering, particularly among the disadvantaged in our society. The homeless and the inhabitants of common lodging houses represent the very bottom end of society.

Even today, large numbers of homeless people experience difficulty in obtaining medical care, and because they have no fixed address they are often not registered with a general practitioner. Severe underuse of conventional health care facilities by this group is endemic (Maclean and Naumann 1979).

Providing health care for the homeless is difficult: many general practitioners are reluctant to register patients of no fixed abode, and many hospital specialities deny responsibility for the homeless by invoking catchment area restrictions (British Medical Journal 1989). The Department of Health have acknowledged that arrangements instituted in 1975 to provide for the homeless and rootless have 'not been fully effective'. The medical disorders of the homeless are common illnesses magnified by disordered living conditions. The stress of street life, psychiatric disorders, and sociopathic behaviour patterns obstruct medical intervention and contribute to the chronicity of disease. Recent studies on the health status of homeless persons report that being without a home is associated with excess morbidity and mortality (Brickner et al 1984) and may increase the risk of communicable diseases, injuries, hypothermia and malnutrition, and may worsen existing conditions. Moreover, the homeless may have special problems with access to health care because of poverty, poor education, lack of social skills, and unemployment.

The homeless form a subgroup with a pattern of morbidity different from the general population which, when allied to their adverse social circumstances, means that they require more than the average amount of medical care. For example, Scott et al (1966) revealed that less than half were free from chronic disease and Alstrom et al (1975) reported a significant excess mortality for all age groups. Alcoholism, psychiatric illness, and a high incidence of chronic medical morbidity, especially peptic ulceration, trauma and respiratory disease, including tuberculosis are particularly prevalent amongst this group (Shanks 1981, 1982a, 1984, 1988, 1989). Many of these conditions result in considerable handicaps and are sustained by an extremely poor environment.

More recently the health needs of homeless families as opposed to the single homeless have been highlighted (Golding 1987, Lowry 1989). Many homeless families are from ethnic minorities and some barely speak English. Families who feel that their problems are temporary might also leave registering with a general practitioner until they have organized basic amenities. They may be unfamiliar with local services and some ethnic families are hampered by language difficulties from understanding how to gain access to a general practitioner. Because they live in overcrowded, temporary accommodation they face many health risks. Their children are under-nourished, under-motivated, and frequently infected with diarrhoeal illnesses and chest infections (Thompson 1986). They have low levels of immunization and irregular developmental checks (Boyer 1986), and they frequently require hospital admission (Golding 1987, Victor et al 1989). Damp and mouldy living conditions have an adverse effect on symptomatic ill health, particularly in children (Platt et al 1989) where it leads to higher rates of respiratory symptoms (Martin et al 1987). Homeless women are twice as likely to have problems and three times as likely to be admitted to hospital during pregnancy as other women. Health visitors are presently concerned about the nutrition of such people in bed and breakfast accommodation (Drennan and Stearn 1986) where depression and stress among parents may predispose them to child abuse.

The homeless population comprises a kaleidoscope of people. Recent studies have, nevertheless, shown that homeless people tend to be of Celtic or northern origin, and are usually male, single and unemployed. Homeless people frequently suffer from psychiatric disorders and social ostracism (Shanks 1982b, 1988, 1989). The high prevalence of divorce, separation, or never having married among this population, together with coming from a broken home may be a part of a picture of social and emotional deprivation that started early in life. There are some women who are homeless but little is known about them, partly because they are in a minority. Higgs and Hayward (1910) described the poor working conditions and low wages which faced employed women in early twentieth century Britain. Unwanted pregnancies often forced women into common lodging houses or workhouses, where they existed with prostitutes and the mentally ill. Today, changes in the housing system force many women and single mothers, who rely disproportionately on the dwindling public sector, on to the streets or into short-term insecure lodgings with friends and relatives. Previous studies tend to suggest that there is a higher incidence of homelessness among women in Scotland than in England and Wales. For example, Scott et al (1966) reported that 34 per cent of the inmates of Edinburgh lodging houses were female. In a nationwide survey of hostels and lodging houses Digby (1976) estimated that approximately 2,200 women were living in such conditions compared with 23,300 men. Here, women were found to be more socially stable than men in terms of having a job and contact with relatives, but a contrasting picture was painted by Brandon (1973) who described the first year of a community run for 45 destitute women. The first few months were characterized by overdoses, slashed wrists and suicide. However, by encouraging the residents to take responsibility for the community and by instituting encounter groups, the milieu improved, and some of the residents found a degree of stability.

More recently, in a considerably larger study from Manchester, Shanks (1981) reported 5.6 per cent of the population of homeless hostel users to be female. A mobile surgery for the homeless in London reported only 13 out of 146 persons were female (Ramsden et al 198), and the recent Salvation Army report discovered that 12 per cent of people sleeping rough on the street were female (Canter et al, 1989). In the report *Homeless Single Persons* (National Assistance Board 1966) it was discovered that proportionately fewer of the women were in the middle age group, 55 per cent were English, 27 per cent Scottish, and there was a negligible number of Irish. This is in marked contrast to the homeless male population. Why is there an apparently lower incidence of homelessness among females? Are they institutionalized in mental hospitals, which are known to contain more women than men in this country? Can women more successfully live alone in digs or lodgings, or is women's homelessness more likely to be 'hidden'—when they tolerate violent relationships or seek a succession of unsatisfactory lodgings with relatives—because so few initiatives for homeless people are open to women. Certainly there is substantially less provision for homeless females. In 1965 there were 31,932 beds (92 per cent) in hostels for men and only 2,664 (8 per cent) for women (National Assistance Board 1966). The distribution of beds showed a marked geographical bias with well over half the local authority beds in the north west of England, and a quarter in Scotland. Lodging houses for women do, however, tend to be of a far superior standard than those available to men.

Pregnancy is the leading reason for placement in temporary accommodation in 18 per cent of homeless households in London, 11 per cent in other metropolitan boroughs, and 14 per cent in non-metropolitan boroughs (Audit Commission, 1989). If these figures are applied to the Department of Environments' homeless statistics (1987) then 14,000 (1 in 50) births are to homeless women in England and Wales. Hein (1973) reported on the premature onset of sexual activity among homeless women. Their poor educational status, coupled with a general lack of responsibility and increased promiscuity, resulted in a high incidence of pregnancy. Conway (1988) conducted a survey of homeless women in bed and breakfast accommodation and found that 25 per cent had low birth weight babies (less than 2.5kg). Furthermore they booked in late for antenatal care, were poor attenders at clinics throughout pregnancy, and had more complications such as anemia and infections.

A study of the obstetric outcome of homeless women at St Mary's Hospital, London (Paterson and Roderick 1990) revealed sociodemographic characteristics and obstetric risk factors that would be likely to lend to poorer outcomes in pregnancy. There was a high proportion of women who were young, high parity and of IndoPakistani origin. However, the study was unable to demonstrate any significant differences in the outcome of pregnancy that could be directly attributed to living in bed and breakfast accommodation.

There have been recent enquiries into perinatal and neonatal mortality, in no small measure due to the failure of this country's figures to decline as rapidly as those in the rest of Europe (Committee on Child Health Services 1976). Perinatal death (Balarajan and Botting, 1989) is much more common than maternal death. In 1975, for each maternal death, excluding abortions, there were 175 perinatal deaths (Royal College of General Practitioners 1981). Chalmers and McIlwaine (1980) have proposed setting up a national enquiry system into perinatal mortality. It is well recognized that those in the lower social classes suffer a significantly increased perinatal mortality rate. The perinatal mortality rate of social class V is double that of social class IV, and the provision of health care to the latter socially disadvantaged population is difficult.

Because analysis of disease trends show that the environment is the primary determinant of the state of general health in any population, the results of the outcome of pregnancy in such an underprivileged population are of great interest, especially as they represent the very extreme end of the social class system. The aim of this paper therefore is to describe the experience and outcome of providing antenatal care to a group of homeless white women in Manchester.

Method

A prospective survey was conducted in Manchester on homeless females who became pregnant between September 1978 and September 1981. The sample was drawn from those females who resided in hostels, lodging houses and night shelter accommodation, or who slept rough and attended the doctor who provided medical care to the homeless population of the city, as previously described (Shanks 1983).

All consultations were performed in a room available for medical purposes in a large female municipal common lodging house. Further information regarding past obstetric history, the fate of previous children and relevant medical history was obtained from the general practitioners' notes, social services department, and hospital records.

Results

A total of 43 single, pregnant, caucasian homeless females were seen and monitored over a three year period (Table 10.1). Prior to pregnancy only one was using regular contraception, the pill, and a number considered themselves infertile because they had not fallen pregnant earlier. Three out of the total requested termination of pregnancy and, of the remainder, all except two planned to keep the child. Of the 43 women, 33 (77 per cent) had been married previously. Disturbingly, only 37 (86 per cent) admitted to knowing who the father of their child was, and of the men concerned only two (5 per cent) were employed. Only six (16 per cent) of the fathers provided any support or encouragement throughout the pregnancy.

Of the homeless women studied 36 (84 per cent) had had previous children and 34 (79 per cent) had their first pregnancy at

Table 10.1. *Age of pregnant homeless (1978–81)*

age	numbers	per cent
16–19	16	37
20–24	11	26
25–29	7	16
30–34	5	12
35–39	4	9

the age of seventeen, or less. None of the earlier children were still with the mother. Five (12 per cent) had four children; eight (19 per cent) had three; twelve (28 per cent) had two and eleven (26 per cent) had one, thus providing a total of 79 children separated from their mother and possibly living in neglected, underprivileged circumstances. Of these children, five (6.3 per cent) had died; one anencephalic, two had spina fifida, one died a cot death, and one, aged five, died of pneumonia. Eleven (14 per cent) children had been adopted and the remainder were in local authority care.

All except two of the pregnant women were smokers (95 per cent). Five (12 per cent) smoked between one and ten cigarettes daily; 29 (67 per cent) between ten and twenty, and seven (16 per cent) more than 20 daily. Seventeen (40 per cent) were alcoholics; six (14 per cent) were illicit drug takers, and nine (21 per cent) had a previous history of admissions to psychiatric units for major psychotic illnesses.

Table 10.2 reveals that this group tends to attend for antenatal care late in pregnancy. They proved themselves to be multiple nonattenders at antenatal clinics despite the fact that they frequently suffered complications during the antenatal period. Twenty-nine (67 per cent) had anaemia at first booking; 29 (67 per cent suffered from chronic vaginal infections; and 21 (49 per cent) suffered from urinary tract infection during the antenatal period. Four (9 per cent) had an antepartum haemorrhage.

Eleven (26 per cent) of this sample left the area unexpectedly and were unable to be followed up, including two who had requested termination. The outcome of the remaining pregnancies was satisfactory. All the babies were delivered after 37 weeks gestation and before 42 weeks. There were no stillbirths and no major congenital abnormalities. One child was born with six digits. However, 33 per cent of the babies were less than 2.5 kgs (low

Table 10.2. *Length of gestation when first consulting the doctor (1978–81)*

	number	per cent
8–11 weeks	4	9
12–16 weeks	9	21
17–20 weeks	7	16
> 20 weeks	23	54
Total	43	100

birth weight) and 21 per cent were below 1.5 kg at birth. None of the mothers breast-fed.

Discussion

The group of homeless women included in the Manchester study had experienced deprivation and maladjustment. Pregnancy for this cohort tends to be a Mal rather than a pleasure, and the problems are compounded because such pregnancies are often unplanned.

The Health Visitors Association and the General Medical Services Committee (1989) have recently examined the problem of health care for homeless families. Some of the difficulties faced by homeless pregnant women relate to how health care is provided and procedures aimed at removing financial and organizational barriers that prevent homeless families from gaining access to primary health care should be applauded. The report suggests that each district health authority should have a liaison officer for homeless persons who has the responsibility for informing health visitors about the arrival of a new family, arranging transfer of the relevant notes, and informing the family practitioner committee about the number of people in temporary accommodation.

Maternal and child welfare has long been a cause of concern and particular attention has been focused on teenage mothers (Simms and Smith 1986). In Britain the number of babies born to those aged 15–19 years decreased from 96, 109 in 1966 to 60, 750 in 1984. However, the number of illegitimate babies born to mothers in this age group increased from 22, 305 (23.2 per cent) to 36, 544 (60 per cent (OPCS 1975).

At the end of the 1970s, Townsend (1979) illustrated the range and extent of poverty in the UK using a series of case descriptions, one of which was a single teenage mother living in Glasgow. Unfortunately, little seems to have improved since that time.

(Williams et at 1987). If poverty does influence the health of women and their children, inequalities in health will persist as long as social disadvantage continues. Although pregnant women are supposedly priority cases for allocation of housing, a recent report strongly challenges this (Conway 1988).

Homeless women are twice as likely to have problems and three times as likely to be admitted to hospital during pregnancy as other women. The social problems of homelessness, unemployment, poverty and single parenthood are compounded by a range of behaviour that also proves detrimental to health. A quarter of the babies born to mothers living in bed and breakfast accommodation are of low birth weight compared with the national average of 7 per cent (Conway 1988). In this study 33 per cent of babies born weighed less than 2.5kg and 21 per cent weighed less than 1.5kg. Low birth weight children score badly on scales of children's ability and there is a growing fear that learning difficulties will become increasingly apparent as these children grow up.

The proportion of babies with low birth weight in New York has been increasing since 1984. This has been mainly attributed to cocaine abuse which is known to retard intrauterine growth, and to be a major cause of homelessness in the USA. The number of infants born to drug abusing mothers has trebled since 1981. (American Journal of Public Health 1990). In 1988, 11 per cent of pregnant women in the USA used drugs during pregnancy, and some 375,000 newborns annually may be damaged by drug exposure.

It is of great concern that 14 per cent of the mothers in this study were illicit drug users, 40 per cent were alcoholics, and 95 per cent were smokers. 21 per cent of mothers had a history of previous admission to hospital for a major psychiatric illness. The instances of psychiatric illness amongst the homeless is high, especially among women. (Shanks 1989; Herzberg 1987).

It is conceivable that those dealing with homeless women are prepared to tolerate a greater degree of behavioural disturbance than they would expect from a similar group of men. This explains why homeless women are more likely to have psychiatric illness. It is likely that the police will deal more sympathetically when a women is behaving strangely and initiate a hospital admission whereas in similar circumstances a male is likely to be charged and remanded in prison. Indeed, Herzberg (1987) has shown that homeless women are significantly more likely to be referred to hospital by the police than homeless men. In addition, women admitted from the community are significantly more likely than men to be presented via the emergency clinic rather than organized channels of referral.

It is therefore possible to hypothesize that the women who

become homeless and gain hospital admission are more disturbed group than their male counterparts. Homeless women tend to cooperate poorly with treatment and are significantly more likely to discharge themselves from hospital than men (Herzberg 1987) and be subsequently readmitted (Byers et al 1978). Thus a homeless female who is mentally ill seems to be trapped in a revolving door between hospitalization and homelessness.

The neglect of breast feeding was disturbing because breast feeding is known to confer protection against gastroenteritis in children (Howie et al 1990). This has particular relevance to the homeless as an increase in childhood infections has been reported in bed and breakfast hotels (Conway 1988).

The outcome of pregnancy in homeless women is poor compared with the general population. Antenatal care is an important service designed to monitor and manage the process of pregnancy and allows the early detection and treatment of anaemia or other medical conditions, education about smoking, alcohol and drug abuse, and advice regarding appropriate social security benefits. Antenatal care may be improved by earlier booking, and in this study 54 per cent were booked in after 20 weeks gestation.

There are six sociocultural factors that are consistently related to the amount of antenatal care received:

1 ability to pay;
2 attitude towards the health profession;
3 delay in suspecting pregnancy;
4 delay in telling others about the pregnancy;
5 perception of the importance of antenatal care; and
6 initial attitudes about pregnancy (Poland et at 1987).

These factors should be addressed when considering an improvement in the provision of antenatal care to the homeless, especially since there is good evidence that the mortality of infants in the first four years of life is twice as high among late antenatal attenders. Nevertheless, although antenatal clinics may be freely available, they may be relatively inaccessible to the homeless because of a lack of support, reliance on a dwindling public transport system, differences in values and attitudes, a fear of doctors, illiteracy, a lack of continuity of care, and previous experience of a discourteous service.

Ways to improve access to care throughout pregnancy could include the development of outreach services for 'at risk' women. Information about health services should be clearly displayed in social security offices, hostels and hotels, and areas known to be frequented by such at risk persons.

References

Alstrom C H, Lindelius R, Salum I 1975 Mortality among homeless men. *British Medical Journal*, **70**: 245–252

Audit Commission 1989 *Housing the homeless: the local authority role*. HMSO, London

Balarajan R, Botting B 1989 Perinatal mortality in England and Wales: variations by mother's country of birth (1982–85). *Health Trends*, **121**: 79–84

Beveridge W H 1942 *Social insurance and allied service*. Report by Sir William Beveridge, HMSO, London

Boyer J 1986 Homelessness from a health visitor's viewpoint. *Health Visitor* **59**: 332

Brandon D 1973 Community for homeless women. *Social Work Today*, **4**: 167

Brickner P W, Scharer L K, Conaran B, Elvy A, Savarese M Eds 1985 *Health care of homeless people*. Springer, New York

British Medical Journal 1989 Figures on homelessness. *British Medical Journal* **298**: 210

Byers E S, Cohen S, Harshbarger D D 1978 Impact of after care services on recidivism of mental hospital patients. *Community Mental Health Journal*, **14**: 26–34

Canter D, Drake M, Littler T, Moore J, Stockley D, Ball J 1989 *The faces of homelessness in London*. Interim report to the Salvation Army. Department of Psychology, University of Surrey

Carstairs V, Morris R 1989 Deprivation: explaining differences in mortality between Scotland, England and Wales. *British Medical Journal* **299**: 866–9

Chalmers I, McIlwaine G 1980 *Perinatal audit and surveillance*. Proceedings of the eighth study group of the Royal College of Obstetricians and Gynecologists. Royal College of Obstetricians and Gynecologists, London

Cloake E 1989 Report on confidential enquires into maternal deaths in England and Wales: a summary of the main points. *Health Trends*, **121**: 79–84

Committee on Child Health Services 1976 *Fit for the future* (Court Report). HMSO, London

Conway J 1988 *Prescription for poor health: the crisis of homeless families*. London Food Commission, Maternity Allowance, SHAC. Shelter, London

Department of the Environment 1987 *Homeless Statistics*. HMSO, London

Digby P W 1976 *Hostels and lodging for single people*. HMSO, London

Drennan V, Stearn J 1987 Health visitors and homeless families. *Health Visitor*, **59**: 340

Golding A M B 1987 the health needs of homeless families. *Journal of the Royal College of General Practitioners*, **37**: 433

Health Visitors Association and General Medical Services Committee 1989 *Homeless families and their health*. British Medical Association, London

Hein K 1973 Age at first intercourse among homeless adolescent females. *Journal of Paediatrics* **83**: 6, 147–148

Herzberg J L 1987 No fixed abode: a comparison of men and women admitted to an east London psychiatric hospital. *British Journal of Psychiatry* **150**: 621–627

Higgs M, Hayward E E 1910 *Where shall she live? The homelessness of the women worker*. P S King and Son, London

Howie P W, Forsyth S, Ogston S, Clark A, Florey C V 1990 Protective effect of breast feeding against infection. *British Medical Journal,* **300**: 11–16

Lowry S 1989 Caring for the homeless. *British Medical Journal* **298**: 210

Maclean U, Naumann L 1979 Primary medical care for the single homeless. The Edinburgh experiment *Health Bulletin,* **6**

Marsh G N, Channing D M 1986 Deprivation and health in one general practice. *British Medical Journal* **292**: 1173–76

Martin C J, Platt S, Hunt S M 1987 Housing conditions and ill health. *British Medical Journal,* **294**: 1125

Metcalfe D 1981 Medical care for inner cities. *Lancet* **1**: 731

National Assistance Board. 1966 *Homeless single persons.* HMSO, London

Office of Population Censuses and Surveys 1974 and 1975 *Birth statistics in England and Wales,* HMSO, London

Paterson C M, Roderick P 1990 Obstetric outcome in homeless women. *British Medical Journal* **301**: 263–66

Perinatal Mortality, Surveillance and Audit 1981 Journal of the *Royal College of General Practitioners* **31**: 643

Platt S D 1989 Damp housing, mould growth and symptomatic health state. *British Medical Journal* **298**: 1673

Poland M L, Ager J W, Olson J M 1987 Barriers to receiving adequate prenatal care. *American Journal of Obstetrics and Gynaecology,* 297–303

Ramsden S S , Nyiri P, Bridgewater J, El Kabir D J 1989 A mobile surgery for the single homeless in London. *British Medical Journal* **298**: 372–74

Sargaison E M 1954 *Growing old in common lodgings.* Nuffield Provincial Hospitals Trust, London.

Scott R, Gaskell R G, Morrell D C 1966 Patients who reside in common lodging houses. *British Medical Journal* **2**: 1561–64

Shanks N J 1981 *Demographic features of inmates of common lodging houses.* MSc thesis, University of Manchester

Shanks N J 1982a Medical Care for the homeless. *British Medical Journal* **284**: 1679–80

Shanks N J 1982b Mortality among inmates of common lodging houses. *Journal of the Royal College of General Practitioners* **34** : 540–543

Shanks N J 1983 Medical provision for the homeless in Manchester. *Journal of the Royal College of General Practitioners* **33**: 40–43

Shanks N J, Carroll K B 1984 Persistent tuberculous disease among inmates of common lodging houses. *Journal of Epidemiological and Community Health* **31**: 66–69

Shanks N J 1988 Medical Morbidity of the homeless. *Journal of Epidemiology and Community Health* **12**: 182–185

Shanks N J 1989 Previously diagnosed psychiatric illness among inhabitants of common lodging houses. *Journal of Epidemiology and Community Health* **43**: 375–379

Simms M, Smith C 1986 Teenage mothers and their partners. *A survey in England and Wales*. London, HMSO

Thompson J 1986 Homelessness: a priority for political action, *Health Visitor* **59**: 325

Townsend P 1979 *Poverty in the United Kingdom. A survey of household resources and standards of living* Harmondsworth, Penguin Books.

Victor C R, Connelly J, Roderick P, Cohen C 1989 Use of hospital services by homeless families in an inner London health district. *British Medical Journal* **299**: 725–27

Williams S, Forbes J F, McIlwaine G, Rosenberg K 1987 Poverty and teenage pregnancy. *British Medical Journal*, **294**: 20–21

Winkelstein W 1972 Epidemiological considerations underlying the allocation of health and disease care resources. *International Journal of Epidemiology* **1**: 69–74

11 Special health care needs of families in bed and breakfast accommodation

Jean Conway

Introduction and background

Bed and breakfast hotels have become firmly established as a form of housing. Throughout the last decade English local authorities have never housed fewer than 1,200 households in hotels, and countless other people resort to bed and breakfast as the only kind of accommodation they can find.

Because individual households are not generally expected to spend very long periods in bed and breakfast (though there are many exceptions to this), the problems facing people in this form of accommodation have received scant attention from service providing agencies such as social services, health, and education authorities. Today, however homes in bed and breakfast establishments have become a long term form of housing provision. Because welfare agencies have not recognized this, they do not provide a level of service appropriate to the needs of those who have to live there.

Hotel residents are particularly subject to health risks because conditions in hotels are often very poor and sometimes dangerous. Living in a hotel is stressful and depressing, making residents more prone to poor health. Those who live in hotels tend to be people who cannot afford any better kind of housing, such as the unemployed, those on low wages, large families, and those experiencing language or cultural barriers. Even in normal circumstances, such people are vulnerable to health risks.

To amplify this last point, there is clear evidence of the relationship between poverty and health (Townsend and Davidson 1982; Whitehead 1987; BMA 1982). Diet has been identified as a crucial factor influencing general health status and there are a number of studies which show that the diet of people on low incomes is improving more slowly than that of the population in general (Cole-Hamilton and Lang 1986). Poverty may also mean that people cannot afford adequate heating or clothing, and there is evidence to show that the poor have less access to good health care than the rest of the population (Townsend and Davidson 1982).

Housing acts as a crucial link between poverty and health because, as shown by successive house condition surveys, poor people tend to live in the worst housing (Department of the Environment 1981, 1986). Those who have failed to secure any form of permanent housing, the homeless, are in the worst position of all and are amongst the poorest and most vulnerable in society.

Research outline

A number of studies have documented the problems of those who live in hotels (Randall, Francis and Brougham 1981; Murie and Jeffers 1987). This paper focuses on a study which was specifically designed to examine the needs of homeless hotel residents in relation to health—the full project is outlined in Conway, 1988. This research looked at mothers and children under five years old—a group thought to be particularly at risk. The study was carried out in 1986 and 1987, and had four main elements:

1 Interviews with 57 women who were pregnant or had children under five who had been living in bed and breakfast hotels for several months.
2 A detailed analysis of the diet and eating patterns of the women interviewed.
3 Interviews with a range of professionals who have contact with women and children living in hotels, including health visitors, GPs, midwives, paediatricians and environmental health officers.
4 Examination of health records for pregnant women and children. Data for hotel residents were compared with two control groups of families not living in hotels (from similar socioeconomic and ethnic backgrounds in London, and the general population in Manchester).

169

The findings of this research therefore combine qualitative and quantitative information on the health problems of those living in hotels and highlight a range of issues concerned with the provision of health and welfare services.

The work was carried out in three areas: London, Manchester, and Southend. London has the greatest concentration of families living in hotels. Manchester was included because attempts had been made there to bring together the health and housing services for hotel residents in the city. Southend illustrates another area outside London with a concentration of hotel residents.

Conditions in hotels

Visits to hotels spread across the three towns provide a catalogue of the conditions in which many homeless families have to live. In general the standards and conditions found were appalling. Most households in the survey had to share the WC and the bath or shower. Eleven out of the 57 shared with 10 or more people. For a quarter of the households the WC was on another floor of the hotel, and for a further quarter the bath or shower was also on another floor. In a hotel—where there is little privacy; where it is not safe to leave young children alone in the bedroom; where the room may have to be locked every time it is left; and where there may well be a queue for the WC or bathroom—having no facilities on the same floor is extremely inconvenient and could be dangerous. The women were also very anxious about cleanliness in the hotels. Dirt, smells, fleas and cockroaches were often mentioned. In some hotels the management did not even clean the common areas and the residents had to buy materials and clean the WCs, halls etc. themselves.

People in bed and breakfast hotels generally have financial as well as housing problems. Hotel life is expensive, most of those living in them are unemployed, and those who have jobs tend to have low wages. Yet living in a hotel itself makes it more difficult to get work, and some people in the survey found themselves in an 'unemployment trap' where they would not have been able to live in the hotel if they had taken work. The disposable incomes of those in the study were extremely low and people were having to go without basic necessities. Nearly a third of the women were sometimes going without food. The lack of money is likely to affect the health of hotel residents both by increasing their worries and by restricting their diet.

Overcrowding

While conditions in hotels vary greatly, most would not be comfortable to stay in even for a short period of time. For families with young children who must live there for many months or even years, the most striking problem in this survey was the lack of space. Based on interviewer estimates, over a third of the rooms were thought to be under 110 square feet—the equivalent of a room 10 feet by 11 feet. These were mostly occupied by two people (either a couple or mother and child), but there were five families in the survey where three people had to live in a room of this size. Larger families tended to have larger rooms and some of the very large families had two rooms. However one family with two adults and four children were living in a dark basement room approximately 10 feet by 17 feet; with two double beds pushed together, the sink, wardrobe, and chest of drawers—there was little space left for the possessions of a family of six.

An attempt was made to relate the situation of those in the survey with the statutory definition of overcrowding. Of the 42 households where details were obtained, nearly half were statutorily overcrowded. Of the 110 children of all ages in these families, at least 33 were sharing their bed with another child and 13 had to share with an adult. Some rooms were too small even for a baby's cot. One child just had a mattress on the floor while another had a fold-up bed which, when open, fitted across the doorway.

The high level of overcrowding experienced by many bed and breakfast families is exacerbated by the lack of safety and security many feel in the hotel. There are real fears for young children playing both in halls and stairways and in cramped rooms with kettles and cooking equipment. Open fuse boxes, multiple adaptors, and trailing wires were not uncommon. One family had resorted to putting a wardrobe in front of their insecure fourth floor window to prevent the children from falling out; the small room was in darkness all day. Few women had faith in the fire alarms, where one existed at all. Many also feared the lack of privacy and the fact that strangers had access to the halls and corridors.

All the problems with hotel life found in the survey are made more acute by the fact that many people have to spend long periods of time there and usually do not know when they may be rehoused. The women's general sense of having been dumped in a hotel and forgotten made it harder to cope with the conditions they were having to live in, and it is likely to have increased their stress and anxiety.

Food and cooking

The storage, preparation and cooking of food are all likely to play an important part in determining what kinds of foods can be eaten. Food storage was a major problem for most of the women in the survey. Some hotels did not allow residents to keep any

171

food at all in their rooms and nearly half the women did not have a fridge in their room or elsewhere. Six said they could keep no food at all, including two with babies who felt unable to wean them because of this. The lack of space to prepare food was also a problem and there was particular concern about using knives in the cramped bedrooms where young children could hurt themselves.

Access to kitchens and cooking facilities is crucially important. The Association of London Authorities' code of practice for kitchens suggests that one full set of kitchen facilities should be available for every five people and should not be more than one floor away. (Facilities should include an oven, burners, grill, sink fridge and storage.) Twenty two of the 57 women in this survey had no kitchen they could use at all. This included six who had no means of preparing even a hot drink as there was also no kettle in the bedroom.

Only five had exclusive use of a kitchen. The rest shared a kitchen with at least three other families and many shared with large numbers; in six cases over twenty families had to share the kitchen. One had only six rings for over 20 families while another had just four rings for over 40 families to use. The shared kitchens were often a long way from the bedrooms; two-thirds were two or more floors away, and many of the women were concerned about having to carry hot food or pots and pans up and down the stairs—often with young children in tow. Where there were kettles and cooking facilities in the rooms these were perceived as dangerous.

The survey found that most hotels do not cater for people providing meals for themselves. Some homeless families live in hotels for long periods of time and many are forced to rely on take-aways and cafes. Apart from being very expensive, this has a marked effect on the quality of their diet, as shown below.

Food and diet

The importance of nutrition to long-term and short-term health has been well known for some time. As part of the interviews with women in hotels they were asked what they had to eat and drink the day before. If this was not typical they were asked what was. They were also asked how many times a week they ate 30 different designated foods. The dietician involved in the research was able to assess the diets of 48 of the women. Twenty were eating a 'poor' diet, 24 had 'average' diets while only 4 had 'good' diets. Well over a third had diets which were very high in fat and sugar and low in dietary fibre.

Seven of the women were living primarily on snacks, only occasionally supplemented with a hot meal. In spite of hotel accommodation being generally referred to as 'bed and breakfast', well over half the women never had a hotel breakfast either because none was provided or because it was inconvenient, unsuitable or 'inedible'. There was heavy reliance on take-aways, cafes, snacks and prepackaged convenience foods. Over a third never prepared a cooked meal for their families or did so less than once a week.

The overall quality of the women's diets was affected to a great extent by the availability and cleanliness of a kitchen and food preparation facilities. Those with access to a decent kitchen were much more likely to be eating a better diet than those without. The lack of money was also an important restriction on diet. Nearly a quarter of the women were going without food from time to time because they could not afford it and one in ten said their children sometimes went without food. Money constraints were found to play an even greater part in poor diets in this study than in a comparable study of people with low incomes in the general population, suggesting that living in a hotel accentuates financial problems (Lang et al 1984). Changes to the benefit system introduced in April 1989 have further cut the income of many families in bed and breakfast hotels.

The women expressed grave concerns about the poor quality of their diets and the expense. The less able they were to cater for themselves—the more they worried. They were particularly anxious about the fact that they could not give their children the kind of food they knew they should have. These concerns were reflected by the health visitors. One health visitor in Manchester felt that the diet 'almost amounts to malnutrition standards in some cases'. Since this research was carried out there have been changes to the benefit system which leave families in hotels with even less money to spend on food—in some cases as little as £1 per person a day. It is reasonable to assume that their already inadequate diets are now even poorer.

Women's health and housing

It is generally accepted that, on the whole, women are more affected by their home environment than are men. This is partly because they are more exposed to that environment. Women tend to spend more time in the home caring for children and old or infirm relations. Because women bear the main responsibility for child care they tend also to be more concerned and involved when children are ill. Because women generally earn less than men and have less economic independence they have less spending power and less opportunity to go outside the home. Women are also less mobile than men: fewer drive or have access to a car and some fear public transport and the streets, especially at night.

Women's greater exposure to the home environment means that they receive relatively high 'doses' of unhealthy dwellings in settings where damp, cold, mould, and overcrowding are the norm. The adverse health effects of living in high rise flats has also been documented. Women bringing up young children in high rise flats suffer problems of isolation and anxieties about children's safety and their play needs (Littlewood and Tinker 1981). These kinds of problem are compounded for single mothers. Forty per cent of households accepted as homeless by local authorities in Britain are single parents, and the vast majority of these are women. The study of the health effects of living in hotels therefore focused specifically on women.

Women's health

> Sheila and her fourteen-month-old daughter live in a room approximately 7 feet by 15 feet. The small window is at least 6 feet high up on the wall and gives very little light. As there is no room for a cot, the daughter shares Sheila's bed and disturbs her through the night. The hotel has no kitchen and food is not allowed in the rooms. Sheila does not even have a kettle to make a hot drink. She is often hungry, but worries more about her daughter who is often ill and does not seem to be growing.

Given situations like the above, found in the survey, it is not surprising that one of the most striking findings was the degree of stress experienced by the women. Tension manifested itself in a number of ways: two women felt that they were very close to battering their children; two had started to drink heavily; one was losing weight rapidly despite the fact that she was still breast feeding her baby. Many experienced severe depression and some had started to take pills to help.

Boredom, isolation and loneliness were important factors undermining the mothers' quality of life. Nearly half the women in the survey, especially those with larger families, said they normally spent at least eight hours during the day in their bedroom, often not going out of the room at all except to the WC or bathroom. Many, especially those in London, were also isolated because they had been placed in hotels far from their own area.

In response to questions about health problems, the most frequently mentioned ailments were severe headaches or migraines. Common also were diarrhoea and chest infections. Many said they generally felt run down and tired and were more susceptible to coughs and colds. Those normally confined in their rooms for eight or more hours during the day were much more likely to have been ill than those who were normally out more. GPs and health visitors were extremely concerned about both the physical and mental health of women in hotels. One London GP saw the main problem as 'a pervasive sense of hopelessness, depression and despair. What you see are subtle changes in their health—more chest infections, more headaches and more anxiety'.

Pregnant women

About one in 50 women having babies each year are homeless and accepted by local authorities. Having experienced the distress of being homeless, a high proportion are then placed in temporary accommodation, and this often takes the form of a hotel. Many are not given a permanent home until after the baby is born.

When women are pregnant, their health is of particular importance. This is well illustrated by Nigel Shanks (Chapter 10, this volume). Pregnant women are generally encouraged to eat well, take care of their health and relax. However, life in a hotel in the kinds of setting described above make such advice impossible to follow. The difficulties of getting proper meals, the stress of living in a noisy overcrowded dwelling, and so on, can enhance the risks associated with pregnancy and negate the pleasures of motherhood. The health of pregnant women in hotels is therefore a major cause for concern, and this study found that such accommodation posed a grave risk to the health and welfare of the mothers and their babies.

The research looked in particular at pregnant women living in hotels. Nineteen of the women in the survey had had babies while living in bed and breakfast and eight were pregnant at the time of the interview. Half said they had had problems during the pregnancy. These included high blood pressure which the doctor had attributed to the stress of living in a hotel, and weight loss in one woman who had been unable to get proper meals. Another woman, finding it hard to walk in the later stages of her pregnancy, often could not get to the kitchen which was two floors away from her bedroom. For one, smoking had been a major problem, because she had been too stressed to give up, in spite of having given up smoking during two previous pregnancies when she had not been living in a hotel.

A good diet is crucially important for a pregnant woman, yet hotel life often makes it very difficult to achieve an adequate diet. The story of one of the pregnant women in the survey highlights the problem. She was seven and a half months pregnant at the time of the interview. She attended college and had to leave in the morning before the time when the hotel breakfast was served. Lunch was usually her first food of the day and she could only afford to buy snack food such as chips or a sandwich. The hotel provided no cooking facilities of any kind for the residents. There was nowhere for storing food and milk could not be kept overnight in the heat of the bedroom. As a vegetarian she had a very limited choice from the local take-aways so her evening meal during the week normally consisted of chips and a milk shake with an occasional pizza. Sometimes she just had biscuits and bread in the evenings. She did not even have a kettle in her room. She only had hot meals at weekends when she returned to her family in another part of London. This woman was desperately worried about her unborn baby because the doctors had told her that the baby's health was affected by her bad diet. She said 'I don't mind if I die, but if my baby dies what will I do?'

The midwives interviewed for the study were extremely concerned about pregnant women in hotels and their babies. These women are often late booking into hospitals and have poor attendance at antenatal classes. Those who have booked into a hospital in their local area often do not change to another hospital near the hotel because they do not know how long they will be living there or where they will move to next. The information collected from health records on problems during pregnancy and labour proved these fears to be well founded. There was a striking difference between those women who were in bed and breakfast during pregnancy and those who moved in after the birth of their baby. Those who were homeless in pregnancy were more than twice as likely to have problems recorded and were more than three times as likely to have been admitted to hospital during the pregnancy. In particular a higher incidence of anaemia was found, and more infections. While hotel life jeopardizes the health of all residents, pregnant women and their babies are especially at risk.

Health of newborn babies in hotels

Birthweight is probably the single most important indicator of a baby's future health. Analysis of the health records for this study shows that, although the number of cases is small, about a quarter of babies born in bed and breakfast hotels have a low birthweight. This is considerably higher than the national average of 7 per cent with a low birthweight. Those born in hotels include a high proportion with Bangladeshi, Indian and Pakistani surnames; yet the incidence of low birthweight in hotel babies is still significantly higher than that for these groups in the general population.

Five out of the 19 babies in the interview survey born while their mothers were living in a hotel were premature, including two with a low birthweight. Altogether five of these 19 babies had not been healthy at birth and two had stayed in hospital for over 10 days. Health professionals, aware of the poor conditions in many hotels, often try to keep newborn babies in hospital longer when the mother lives in a hotel. Nevertheless the mother must eventually cope with the physical and mental stresses of introducing a tiny baby to a cramped room, often several flights upstairs, in a noisy hotel.

Children's health and diet

There were 71 children under five years old in the survey of homeless women, as well as 39 older children. Nearly half of the under fives had suffered from diarrhoea and sickness since living in a hotel, and over a third had been getting chest infections—a higher incidence than would normally be expected. Infections seemed to pass quickly from one child to another and many women said that coughs and could were almost constant amongst the children. Five mothers said their children had developed skin problems since moving to a hotel and several felt that their health problems resulted from their poor diet. One woman who had no access to a kitchen, no kettle, and was not supposed to keep any food in the room, secretly kept some cereal for her eighteen month old daughter and mixed it with hot water from the basin tap to feed her child.

Not only did the hotel children's physical health seem to suffer, but both the mothers and the health professionals identified behaviour problems and slow development. Several children had become regular bedwetters (in one case the child shared the bed with her mother) and over half were felt by their mothers to have become very bad sleepers for their age. Some had become unusually aggressive or active; one would always scream for long periods when returning to the hotel after a trip out. The health professionals also saw a direct link between the accommodation and the slow development of many of the hotel children. They blamed late walking, late talking, late potty training, and speech delays on the restrictions of hotel life.

These restrictions are often imposed because of the dangers present in a hotel, with kettles and cooking equipment in bedrooms, and often no safe place for knives, razors, disinfectant etc. During the interviews it emerged that 22 children had had some kind of accident. These included falling downstairs while playing, burns, and drinking disinfectant. One health visitor described how a one year old had received extensive third degree burns when her mother spilt a pot of hot water over her while carrying the child and the pot up from the basement kitchen to the bedroom. Children

177

either have to spend long periods of time confined to the cramped bedroom, or play in the halls and corridors which are neither safe nor suitable. Some babies are left in their cots or strapped into high chairs or push chairs for long periods to keep them from danger.

Mothers were especially concerned about their children's diet and were distressed that they could not give their children the food they wanted them to have. However the poor diet of the mothers themselves often forces them to give up breastfeeding and rely on bottles for young babies which, in a hotel, carries a grave risk of infection.

Access to health care

In spite of being a high risk group, the survey found that many hotel residents have difficulty getting primary health care and few are getting the extra level of support which may be needed. Looking at developmental tests for young children, the examination of health records shows that, of those babies who moved into bed and breakfast soon after being born, over half missed the six week test which is so crucial for identifying any early problems or handicap. A higher proportion (12 per cent) of those whose mothers had been living in a hotel before the birth had had this test (this is close to the proportion in the control group in London of families from a similar background, but much lower than for the general population in Manchester). However both groups of hotel children tended to miss subsequent developmental checks more often than those not living in hotels. In general more children in hotels also missed immunizations and vaccinations than children not living in hotels.

The study also highlighted serious difficulties with access to GPs. Of the 57 women in the survey, 23 were still with the doctor they had prior to moving to a hotel, 13 had permanently registered with a doctor nearer the hotel, and 19 were temporarily registered locally; two had no GP at all. Half the children under five were only temporarily registered. Some women preferred to stay with their original doctor although they were currently living some distance away. However 14 of the 39 women in London had tried to register with a GP nearer the hotel and had found difficulty in doing so. Three of the 18 women in Manchester and Southend had also had problems. In one case a woman had tried five different GPs before finding one who would take her. The Bangladeshi women in the survey seemed to have particular problems finding a local doctor because they had been placed in a hotel far away from their own community and could not find a Bengali speaking doctor near the hotel. Several health visitors in the study felt that there was a lack of concern shown by some GPs. It is feared that changes to GPs contracts may make some even less inclined to accept homeless people onto their lists. In recognition of this, Lord Ennals sought to introduce a clause into the *National Health Service and Community Care Bill* during its passage through the House of Lords in Spring 1990. This clause would have given homeless people a statutory right to register with a doctor. The proposal was defeated.

Because of the poor and crowded conditions in most hotels, the need for health visitors is especially acute. Yet only 14 of the 46 children under three years old in the survey had a health visitor who came to see them regularly; 22 had a visit only sometimes or just once, and eight had never had a visit at all.

Response of the health services

Some attempts are being made by the health services to bring a better service to homeless families. In Bayswater, London the Family Practitioner Committee will allocate a GP to see a homeless person where there have been difficulties registering. Manchester City Council has appointed a specialist in community medicine who contacts the FPC where there are problems. In Finsbury Park, London one GP has been designated as having 'special interest in homelessness' and has been able to promote better access to services. The Health Visitors Association and the British Medical Association are now working together to improve health care for hotel families, developing practical ideas to improve primary services.

The problem of poor antenatal care has been recognized and addressed by one Manchester hospital. Here pregnant women are allowed to book into the clinic even if they have no letter from a GP; such a letter is usually required before the hospital service can be mobilized, but in the case of homeless women this requirement tends to act as a barrier to access to hospital care.

Health visitors are often in a unique position to identify the health problems arising from hotel life. In areas with high concentrations of bed and breakfast hotels, health visitors often work exclusively with homeless families. However their caseloads are enormous: in London, Southend and Manchester health visitors often have 120–150 homeless families each. Some can only deal with those who have been placed in hotels by the local authority and are not able to work with other families in hotels.

Health visitors and midwives often do not receive adequate information about homeless families placed in hotels in their area.

In many places, particularly London, families are often placed in hotels outside the area of the local authority which has accepted them as homeless and there is no contact between the local authority and the health authority in the receiving area. The Association of London Authorities/London Boroughs Association code of practice on the use of hotels includes procedures for notification, yet the health visitors found the system did not work.

In Finsbury Park a 'health mobile' van has been introduced. It visits the area where hotels are concentrated and is staffed by a Bangladeshi health worker, two health visitors, and a GP. In Bayswater the idea of providing such a basic form of primary care has been rejected, but attempts have been made by the health service to link into other support networks including the playgroup which caters for homeless people.

There are mixed feelings about the provision of specialist services for the homeless. It ensures that services are geared to those in need and the workers have a good understanding of the issues. On the other hand working with the homeless is extremely stressful. It is argued that the existence of separate specialist services marginalises the homeless and the general service may then ignore their needs. There is also the danger that specialist services become second class services. These issues have been discussed in most detail in relation to single homeless people and there has been little debate in relation to specialist services for families (Stern and Stillwell, Chapter 13, this volume; Williams and Allen, 1990 and Chapter 14, this volume).

Response of housing services

The Association of London Authorities and London Boroughs Association have developed a code of practice on the use of hotels and the Bed and Breakfast Information Exchange has been set up in London to coordinate the actions of the boroughs. The success of these initiatives has been restricted by the enormous scale of the problem.

The most significant development over the last few years has been the increased use of other forms of temporary accommodation for the homeless, particularly private sector leasing schemes whereby local authorities lease empty private properties to let on a temporary basis to those accepted as homeless. There are currently about equal numbers placed in hotels and in private leased homes in London—about 7,000 families in each. It is expected that by the beginning of 1990 there will be more in privately leased homes than in bed and breakfast hotels in the capital.

Standards in the privately leased homes are generally far higher than in hotels and residents have exclusive use of facilities including kitchens. However some of the health problems associated with being homeless remain. The use of these schemes is fragmented and notification to other services such as health visitors and midwives is even more difficult than where hotels are used. While many authorities were able to place an increasing proportion of the homeless in hotels in the local area, leased homes are more scattered and many have to move long distances, thus severing their local ties. This means losing support networks and changing GP. Some problems have also arisen concerning responsibility for controlling the scheme and dealing with conditions in the properties.

The most serious concern is that under current Government rules the leases cannot be renewed after three years. This means that within the next two years very large numbers of homeless families will once again need to be found some kind of short term accommodation.

Integrating the services

One of the key issues to emerge from this study is the need to coordinate and integrate services: housing, environmental health, health, social services, and education, in particular. The administrative frameworks within which services operate often act as barriers to improving links between planning and delivery of different services (Spicker 1989). Normal working practices often mean that there is no contact between people in different agencies who work with the same families in the same hotels.

These links need to be made at all levels. In some areas it has been extremely valuable simply to arrange a meeting between homeless families officers, health visitors and social workers, to discuss specific issues concerning particular families or hotels. For example, over a long period of time one hotel manager in London had frequently refused to let health visitors enter the hotel. After the first ever meeting between the health visitors and local authority homelessness officers, a homelessness officer phoned the hotel manager and arranged free access from that day.

At a more formal level, local authorities should take the responsibility for establishing coordinating groups which bring together all the relevant agencies including voluntary and community groups and representatives for the homeless people themselves. The relevant workers should be represented including health visitors, midwives, GPs, public health physicians, community dieticians, environmental health officers, social workers, psychiatric health and social workers, education welfare officers, teachers and housing department staff.

The tasks of such a group might include establishing an efficient system for notifying all relevant people about the placement of families in hotels. It might also develop standards of provision and management for hotel settings and play a role in coordinating training for those who work with homelessness families. The group could ensure proper access to interpreters where needed, and could oversee the planning and monitoring of services. With the increasing number of homeless families living for long periods in temporary accommodation local authorities can no longer rely on *ad hoc* arrangements but need to set up formal procedures to ensure that the provision of services is appropriate and coordinated.

Conclusion

The study described above shows that the health of pregnant women, mothers, and young children who live in hotels is badly affected. This is partly because the conditions in hotels are so poor and totally unsuitable for families. It is also the result of the stress of being homeless and not knowing when they are likely to be rehoused, or where. The fact that many homeless families are placed in hotels far from their original area adds to their vulnerabilty. Both housing and health authorities are providing a totally inadequate level of support to meet their needs. A lot of effort has recently been made to secure other types of temporary accommodation for the homeless which provides considerably better conditions. However there are still major problems and the families' health is still at risk.

Authorities have not responded to the fact that large amounts of temporary accommodation have been used for many years and have become a long term feature of the housing system. While the ultimate solution is, obviously, for there to be more permanent housing, authorities should now pay serious attention to the needs of the thousands of families who will continue to live in inadequate accommodation for the forseeable future.

Reference

British Medical Association 1982 *Deprivation and ill health.* London, BMA Board of Science and Education Discussion Paper

Cole-Hamilton I, Lang T 1986 *Tightening belts: a report on the impact of poverty on food.* The London Food Commission, London

Conway J Ed 1988 *Prescription for poor health: the crisis for homeless families,* SHAC, London

Department of the Environment 1981, 1986 *English house condition survey,* HMSO, London

Lang T et al 1984 Jam tomorrow? Manchester Polytechnic Food Policy Unit, Manchester

Littlewood J, Tinker A 1981 *Families in flats.* HMSO, London

Murie A, Jeffers S. eds 1987 *Living in bed and breakfast: the experience of homelessness in London.* Working paper no. **71**, School for Advanced Urban Studies, Bristol

Randall G, Francis D, Brougham C 1981 *A place for the family.* SHAC, London

Spicker P 1989 *Social housing and the social services.* Longman, London

Townsend P, Davidson N 1982 *Inequalities in health: The Black Report.* Pelican edition, Penguin Books, Harmondsworth

Whitehead M 1987 *The health divide: inequalities in health in the 1980's.* Health Education Council, London

Williams S, Allen I 1990 *Health care for single homeless people,* Policy Studies Institute, London.

12 Approaches to medical care of homeless people in central London

Simon Ramsden

Introduction

The term 'single homeless' encompasses a large and diverse group of people on the margins of our society, grouped together largely because they sleep out or live in temporary or hostel accommodation and are without close family ties. Any attempt to understand or care for homeless people must recognize this diversity. An idea of the types of individuals who make up the single homeless is shown by the classification of Fisher and Breakey (1986) who suggest four broad categories:

1 chronic mentally ill;
2 street people, both male and female, including the so-called 'bag-ladies' who seem to elect for a street existence, shunning all shelter and company;
3 chronic alcoholics who tend to be male and over 45 years of age; and
4 situationally distressed who are less likely to be mentally ill and include many young and new homeless.

Recent domestic strife, loss of a supportive relative, or unemployment are often precipitating factors. Others have devised systems based on mobility and means of support (Mouren et al, 1977). Our own experience of those sleeping out shows that many remain 'roofless' for long periods, rejecting help from day centres or hostels while others at the same site move frequently between hostels, day centres, and a street existence. One theme does, however, unite single homeless people, that of frequent and severe illness. In this paper I would like to describe the ways in which our practice and others have attempted to provide health care to such a varied and needy population.

As we might expect from the description above, the use of health care facilities by the homeless is different from the general population. They are less likely to be registered with a GP and often use casualty departments to obtain primary care. When ill they may not even choose to see a doctor. There are many reasons underlying this pattern, and an understanding of them is vital to both planning appropriate services and appreciating the response of the homeless during medical treatment. Broadly speaking, the reasons underlying this depend on the operation of health care services as they exist at present and the make-up, expectations and life style of the homeless individuals themselves.

General practice clinics have been held in hostels and day centres for many years. Laidlaw (1956) in the 1950s and Scott et al (1966) in the 1960s describe in vivid detail examples of these clinics. A striking theme is the high level of chronic illness encountered, Scott et al (1966) reporting more than 50 per cent. Hostels vary greatly in their makeup and turnover. Some, with many severely mentally or physically ill patients, are very demanding of a general practitioner's time. In contrast Shanks (1988) describes a hostel where the workload, as measured by consultation rates, is slightly below that expected. Mental illness is particularly common, and is a frequent cause of consultation. Recent evidence suggests that the problem is increasing, and that the proportion of mentally ill in hostels is growing, perhaps in part due to the policy of closing long-stay psychiatric hostels (Marshall 1989).

Conventional general practice has for many years cared for many homeless patients. There are limitations as to what this form of health care can handle. For example the actively psychotic and chronic alcoholic patients are sometimes very disruptive and unruly. However, general practice can offer high quality health care and this is to be encouraged.

Many single homeless do not register with GPs. Their mobile lives militate against continuity and future plans. Indeed, when we asked why the homeless people whom we saw on a mobile surgery for those sleeping out had not registered, most answered that they were not ill. Behind this there may often be deeper reasons, related to a sense of inner guilt and fear. One patient, when asked why he had waited so long to consult replied 'because we're afraid of what you might find' (Ramsden et al 1989). Given these limitations to comprehensive health care it is not surprising that accident and emergency departments shoulder the burden of primary health care for many homeless people. The departments usually feel this to be a misuse of their skills (Davidson et al 1983). It is encouraging to note that when primary health care for the homeless was developed in Edinburgh, the use of an accident and emergency department fell and the 'appropriateness' of consultations in the department rose (Powell 1987).

Great Chapel Street Medical Centre

In the 1970s appreciation grew of the problems of the young homeless in the inner cities, particularly London. Great Chapel Street Medical Centre was set up by the Department of Health and Social Security in 1977 for the young homeless, allowing open access primary health care (El-Kabir 1982). The centre was initially open five days a week, staffed by an administrator and nurse with the GP attending for two sessions a week (now increased to five). The numbers of patients attending rapidly rose and now over 1,600 new patients are seen annually. The problems presented by our patients soon began to shape the way the clinic developed. General practitioners have always recognized that illness cannot be separated from the psychological state and the environment of the patient. With the homeless these influences are acutely felt. For most, bronchitis or 'flu' may only be annoying or short term illnesses but in the context of being homeless they may be serious and debilitating. The frequent chronic diseases such as musculoskeletal disease, chronic airways disease and epilepsy are difficult to cope with when a person is homeless and all diminish the ability of patients to care for themselves. Physical disorder is often compounded by mental illness or alcoholism. Many patients, are also suspicious of authority of doctors, as we described, and reluctant to consult. We find that when patients present themselves at the clinic, illness is severe and needs immediate attention. Treatment has to be seen in terms of engaging the patient, developing trust, and then addressing as many of the difficulties as possible or that the patient will allow. Occasionally patients, are seen a number of times before they will feel able to express their fears and allow the doctor to use appropriate treatment or investigation such as radiology. Accommodation and support can only be arranged with true consent and this may not be what the patient wants. However, with further illness, choices change and the *rapport* developed earlier allows patients to choose options that previously were not considered.

In terms of organization, the role of the clinic administrator evolved from that of a receptionist to a central co-ordinating figure. He interviews the patients first, assessing their problems and directing each patient to the doctor, nurse, psychiatrist, or chiropodist as appropriate. He also liaises with housing and social agencies and contacts hospitals or GPs for confirmation and clarification of medical histories. This should ideally be done before the patient consults the doctor. Such an approach allows a rapid and informed response to a patients' problem, addressing not only their medical but also their psychological and social needs.

We found that the range of services needed to be expanded to meet the particular spectrum of problems. In addition to often serious medical conditions, many patients were mentally ill. Schizophrenia and alcoholism are particularly common. In 1984 a senior registrar in psychiatry began a weekly open access session, patients being referred usually by the GP and some through other agencies such as social work departments or probation services. This proved to be highly successful and in 1989 we were able to establish the post of full-time psychiatrist for the homeless at consultant level. There are now four psychiatric sessions a week, with registrars in training providing two clinics. Around 20 per cent of all patients consult the psychiatrist. Schizophrenia is the commonest disorder at 24 per cent with personality disorder, neurosis, and alcohol abuse accounting for the majority of the other disorders.Twenty per cent of the psychiatric patients are sleeping out and 60 per cent reside in local hostels. Despite these circumstances many patients improve substantially and can then go to more suitable and long-term housing.

This model of drop-in medical care seems to be effective in engaging the more 'difficult-to-reach' homeless. Many have been under psychiatric care but are lost to follow-up. Underlying reasons for this include mental deterioration leading to inability to cope with their accommodation, or the relatively rigid times of clinic attendance required for hospital follow up. Some move out of the strict area of their original hospital without new psychiatric care being arranged. Our open access policy with its flexibility circumvents many of these problems. Patients also seem to feel less of a stigma attached to seeing a psychiatrist when this is at the same site as their GP, perhaps feeling that some of the trust invested in the clinic can be transferred to the psychiatrist who works with their own doctor. In an analysis of the clinic we found that those who were most likely to reattend were schizophrenics, including those who had been lost to follow-up by previous psychiatric care (Joseph et al 1990). The clinic seems to be particularly well accepted by these patients. This is particularly encouraging in the light of research by Priest (1976) that showed that although schizophrenia was present in about a quarter of common lodging residents, only 14 per cent of those presenting themselves to psychiatric services were schizophrenic. Patients with personality disorder or alcoholism were overrepresented among those seeing psychiatrists. It is likely that this is in large part due to the ease of access to the clinic, its link with the patient's GP and the attitudes of the staff.

The description above outlines the ways in which the clinic has developed to meet the needs of the homeless. It is highly evolved allowing successful and immediate treatment of the physical, psychiatric and social needs of the patients. The medical care we offer is sensitive to the individual and the assessment of the wishes and capabilities of each patient is of pivotal importance. Homeless patients are frequently suspicious of perceived authority and may expect very little from doctors. The pattern of the clinic described above allows easy access to medical care but what sustains follow-up and compliance with treatment is much more determined by the attitudes and empathy of the staff. An ability to understand and accept the complex mixture of illness, fear and fragility of the patients is quickly perceived by patients. The trust that this can engender is the most powerful influence on the outcome of consultations. This approach demands much from those caring for the patients. The doctor's personal resources are as much a therapeutic instrument as his drugs, though he may find it difficult if this approach does not come easily (Balint 1957). The doctor has to be open and clear with the patient without recourse to the potentially limiting and rigid conventional doctor–patient relationship which the patient would quickly sense and which might lead them to withdraw from any dialogue. An elegant illustration of the importance of *rapport* in the relationship with homeless patients is provided by a paper by Shanks (1981). In this study he compared the consistency of sociodemographic and other data given by samples of homeless to either their GP or someone who introduced themselves as a 'research worker'. The same data were collected six months later from the same patients by the same interviewer. The data given to the GP showed 0.2 per cent inconsistency, whereas that given to the research worker was 39 per cent inconsistent. The influence of the trust and *rapport* given to the doctor is strikingly evident.

The possible outcomes of this type of medicine are much greater than is often the case in more conventional general practice. Illness and incapacity may be the spur to a patient reassessing their lifestyle; clearly severe leg ulceration or respiratory illness may be impossible to improve when living on the streets despite medical and nursing care. However, treatment and social support, including housing, have to be acceptable to the patient. There is often a considerable suspicion of attempts to alter lifestyle and circumstances. Unsolicited attempts by a professional may well be perceived as coercive and obtrusive. Without an empathy for the patient's dilemma and resources, what is desirable to the doctor may well take precedent over what is possible for the patient. Housing and support can be organized from the clinic, but there needs to be careful assessment of the type of housing that will suit patients best. As examples, some alcoholics will cope best with dry houses where there is much support from staff, but others cannot tolerate regulations or what may be felt to be emotional intrusion from others. Such individuals fare far better in larger hostels where rules are minimal and some drinking is permitted. Both types of patient stay only a short time if placed in the wrong environment.

Wytham Hall Sick Bay

Despite the comprehensive and innovative approach outlined above we frequently find that some medical problems are difficult to treat when the patient remains homeless. Chronic leg ulcers and infectious disease require shelter and adequate nutrition to maximise the chances of recovery, in addition to nursing and medical care. The psychiatrically unwell need the stability of an in-patient stay, away from the pressures of a homeless existence. The limitations of treatment for particular conditions are illustrated by tuberculosis, which required consistent compliance with therapy for at least six months to be cured. The results of tuberculosis treatment for homeless patients are particularly poor. Our own research showed that a group of 25 homeless patients with tuberculosis, only a third were cured one year after diagnosis (Ramdsen et al 1988). This reflects the inflexibility of usual medical care and the low priority that many homeless people give to health, in part due to other needs, such as finding a safe place to sleep or obtaining food. Suitable housing is often not available at short notice and may not be ideal when the patient is acutely unwell, as a high degree of medical care is likely to be needed. Unfortunately hospitals cannot provide the answer in many cases. Even if a homeless patient agrees to be admitted, they frequently discharge themselves against advice, finding the authoritarian atmosphere awkward and the restrictions on their lifestyle intolerable.

In 1984 we found a sick bay for the homeless. This is a large house in Maida Vale, the ground floor of which has been converted into a ten bedded residential care home where a bed and three meals a day are provided. It is run by doctors and medical students on a voluntary basis and there is a full-time administrator. All these staff have bed-sits on the premises. Over 750 patients have been admitted, the average length of stay now being around three weeks. Figure 12.1 illustrates the morbidity profile of the patients.

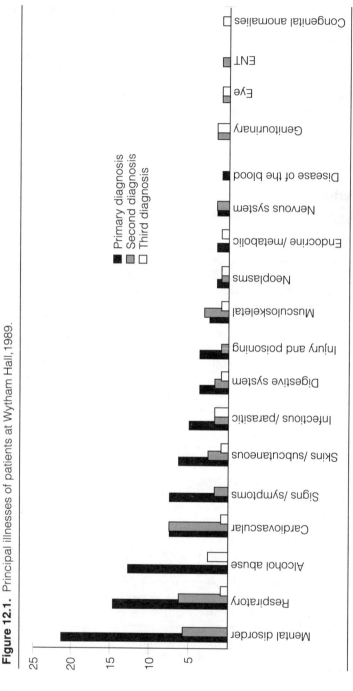

Figure 12.1. Principal illnesses of patients at Wytham Hall, 1989.

It is notable that mental disorder is the most frequent cause of admission, but alcohol abuse is also common, particularly as a secondary complicating factor. Many patients suffer serious illness, such as uncontrolled psychosis, tuberculosis, or severe cardiovascular disease. Many refuse hospital admission but we have developed close links with the local hospitals allowing excellent access to consultant advice and high technology procedures. Rules are minimal: reasonable behaviour; no alcohol; and returning by 7pm. The strength of the sick bay, continuing the trust and *rapport* developed earlier. Management plans evolve as we see how the patients respond, both to the treatment and the new environment. The stay is in some ways a period of grace from the pressures of their usual life, which allows many patients to reassess the direction of their lives. Decisions are made by the patients about their health and future which would have seemed impossible when seen in the clinic.

All patients are housed on discharge, the type of accommodation being carefully matched to the individual. Our major problem in this respect is simply the lack of available housing, particularly supportive housing that can care for fragile and vulnerable patients. Bed and breakfast accommodation is difficult for homeless patients to obtain as landlords are reluctant to accept them, and when obtained is usually less than satisfactory. Rooms are often tiny, and residents must be out early in the morning, the location may be far from areas that the patient knows. Patients normally require continued social support in order to cope, which is arranged before discharge. Around 25 per cent of patients at the sick bay self-discharge, or insist on returning to the streets usually to return to alcohol, a figure which is probably quite good considering the temperaments of many who are admitted. Patients are followed up when necessary by the administrator to ensure that social arrangements are taken up. We recently started to analyse the length of time patients maintain housing after discharge. Early results indicate that after six months about a third remain in self-contained accommodation. The patients that go to this type of housing are usually the most psychiatrically vulnerable. Sixty per cent remain in high quality hostel accommodation and 83 per cent in bed and breakfast accommodation, reflecting the high level of support that is organized. Medical follow-up is usually at our clinics, or, if out of our area, arrangements are made to be registered with a local GP. We see about 80 per cent of patients after discharge at the clinics, or when they return to visit the sick bay.

Mobile surgery

In attempting to reach homeless people a wide range of sites have been used to provide care, including general practice surgeries, hostels, day centres and drop-in clinics. However, many homeless sleep rough and may not use these facilities. In 1987 we began to operate a mobile surgery which visits sites in London where the homeless who sleep out congregate. The vehicle is a Renault Master van converted into a consulting room. The surgery was quickly accepted and up to 25 patients are seen on a single visit.

The results of an analysis of the project are particularly interesting as they again emphasize the diversity of homeless people and the difficulties in providing a comprehensive approach to medical care. The illnesses encountered are typical of a single homeless population. Musculoskeletal, respiratory and skin disorders are most common; alcohol abuse and infestation were also common. What is perhaps very telling is that psychiatric illness was only rarely a presenting problem despite being very obviously common. In many ways the community accepted highly deviant behaviour which no longer became perceived as a problem; this isolated subculture might well be a sanctuary for many psychiatrically unwell, an observation which is probably also true of the large common lodging houses. About a third claimed to never, or rarely, use hostels or day centres and over half had no London GP. The surgery was reaching a particularly isolated subgroup of homeless people. Many had quite severe or disabling illness, but even those with GPs often avoided consulting a doctor, perhaps going to the nearest casualty department when the illness became very severe. This observation on the health behaviour of these people clearly illustrates the inadequacy of using registration with a GP as a measure of the integration of homeless people with conventional health care, or as a marker of the success of out-reach projects, as some have attempted. Of considerable importance is the observation that about a third seen in the mobile surgery at Lincoln's Inn Field consulted at Great Chapel Street Medical Centre within a month of the first consultation (Ramsden et al 1989). This demonstrates that the surgery was able to integrate many of these patients into available health care facilities and adds considerably to the value of the project, as there are obvious limitations to what can be achieved in a single consultation in a mobile surgery. Some patients have to be taken to local casualty departments for possible fractures, others have been admitted directly to our sick bay. Some, however, will still not see doctors in clinics and the mobile surgery is their main source of health care, apart from casualty departments.

Conclusions

The way our practice has evolved since 1977 reflects a number of different pressures and needs. Homeless patients usually present themselves with a combination of medical and psychological problems, often in a state of urgency, compounded by the stresses and conditions of their environment. This requires a multidisciplinary approach, not only in the range of skills available but also in the mind of the doctor. The different resources that have been developed reflect the heterogeneity of homeless people, both in terms of illness and their lifestyles and expectations. An integrated and consistent approach is of pivotal importance in the way our clinics, sick bay and mobile surgery function.

The role of housing, both in respect of homelessness causing ill health, and housing being a means of improving it, is clearly felt. However a 'prescription of housing' to solve these health problems is far from simple. Change is only possible when the wishes, resources, and frailty of a patient are understood, allowing the potential of the housing to match that of the patient. In this sense, the concept of housing becomes more sophisticated and clearly a range of accommodation is needed to meet the varied needs of this diverse population. In this respect resources are woefully inadequate, with large hostels, and bed and breakfast accommodation being the principal available housing, suitable for some, unacceptable to many.

Homeless people present all of us, doctors, nurses, social workers, health planners, and policy makers, with a challenge. A key to meeting their dilemma is in a recognition of their humanity, warts and all, and the avoidance of simplistic and reductionist thinking that ultimately lets down those it seeks to serve.

References

Balint M 1957 *The doctor, his patient and the illness.* Pitman Medical Publishing Company, London

Davidson A G, Hildey A, Floyer M A 1983 Use and misuse of an accident and emergency department in the east end of London. *Journal of the Royal Society of Medicine* **76**: 37–40

El-Kabir D J 1982 Great Chapel Street medical centre. *British Medical Journal* **284**: 480–81

Fisher P J, Breakey W 1986 Homelessness and mental health: an overview. *International Journal of Mental Health* **14**: 6–41

Joseph P L, Bridgewater J, Ramsden S S, El-Kabir D J 1990 A psychiatric clinic for the single homeless in a primary care setting in inner London. *Psychiatric Bulletin* **14**: 270–71

Laidlaw S I 1956 *Glasgow common lodging houses and the people living in them.* Glasgow Corporation, Glasgow

Marshall M 1989 Collected and neglected: Are Oxford hostels for the homeless filling up with disabled psychiatric patients? *British Medical Journal* **229**: 706–9

Mouren M C, Rajaona F R, Thiebaux M, Tatossian A 1977 Le vagabondage: aspects psychologiques et psychopathologiques. *Annales medico-psychologiques* **135**: 415–47

Powell P V 1987 The use of an accident and emergency department by the single homeless. *Health Bulletin* **45**: 255–62

Priest R G 1976 The homeless person and the psychiatric services: an Edinburgh survey. *British Journal of Psychiatry* **128**: 128–36

Ramsden S S, Baer S, El–Kabir D J 1988 Tuberculosis among central London single homeless. *Journal of the Royal College of Physicians* **22**: 16–17

Ramsden S S, Nyiri P, Bridgewater J, El-Kabir D J 1989 A mobile survey for the single homeless. *British Medical Journal* **298**: 372–74

Scott R, Gaskell P G, Morrellss D C 1966 Patients who reside in common lodging houses. *British Medical Journal* **2**: 1561–64

Shanks N J 1981 Consistency of data collected from inmates of a common lodging house. *Journal of Epidemiology and Community Health* **35**: 133–35

Shanks N J 1988 Medical morbidity among the homeless. *Journal of Epidemiology and Community Health* **42**: 183–86

13 Problems of access and attitude: health care and single homeless people

Rick Stern and Barbara Stilwell

Introduction

This paper develops some of the work and ideas presented in a recent report *From the Margins to the Mainstream: Collaborating in Planning Services with Single Homeless People*. A fuller discussion of a wider range of issues and more detailed presentation of research data concerning access to health care for single homeless people are contained in the full report.

What we hope to do in this paper is to present some possible explanations for the apparent failure of health services to meet the health needs of single homeless people and to examine barriers to access from two perspectives. What factors discourage single homeless people from presenting themselves to health services and, conversely, what are health professionals doing to facilitate access? Finally, we look at how one might effect a change in attitudes and what the implications might be, both in terms of our understanding of the meaning of health as well as in facilitating more effective service delivery.

Access to services

There is increasing evidence to suggest that single homeless people have severe difficulties in gaining access to health services.

Table 13.1. *Use of GPs and hospital beds by single homeless people compared with general population in the UK*

	Visits to GP[a]	Use of Hospital bed[b] %
Sleeping out	0.62	26
Large hostels	1.55	8
Other hostels[c]	1.70	9
Supportive housing projects	3.40	29
Others[d]	2.95	27
Average for all groups	1.99	18
General population	4.00	9

Source: Stern and Stilwell (1989)

Notes:

a Average number of visits to a GP per person in the last year

b Percentage of people who reported an in-patient stay in the last year.

c This includes people staying in hostels for single working people and students.

d This includes people in squats and those staying on a temporary basis with friends and relatives.

Two recent reports (Stern and Stillwell 1989; Williams and Allen 1989) present data from three different inner city areas of London revealing a consistently poor pattern of registration with GPs. Surveys suggest that registration amongst the general 'housed' population, even in inner London, may be as high as 97 per cent (Bone 1984). In comparison, the rate for single homeless people is low. Both samples recently surveyed found an overall level of registration of about 60 per cent while the rate for people sleeping out fell to as low as 27 per cent with hardly any of them being registered in the local area.

The report from West Lambeth provides another useful indicator of access to services which can be directly compared to the general population (OPCS, 1986). Registration gives no indication about the actual use of services, so respondents were asked the number of times they had visited a GP in the last year and whether they had been a hospital in-patient in the same period. The results suggested that in general, single homeless people made half as many visits to their GP, but were twice as likely to use a hospital bed than the general population. Once again, people sleeping out suffered the worst problems of all, being over six times less likely to visit a GP and three times more likely to use a hospital bed than the general population (Table 13.1)

These figures clearly indicate low use of primary care services (GPs) but comparitavely high use of secondary care (hospital beds), suggesting that single homeless people often remain untreated until a problem becomes a crisis.

Barriers to access perceived by single homeless people

The right of GPs to refuse registration to anyone, without being required to justify their decision, makes it difficult for a range of people who are considered 'undesirable' to get on to a GPs list. It has generally been recognized that homeless people, especially those sleeping on the streets, suffer from the expectation that they will be problem patients, both in terms of the reaction of other patients in the waiting room and because of the heavy workload the wide range of non-medical problems may generate.

The low level of registration, however, is not simply the result of people being refused directly, but is due to a number of complex factors. The results both from the PSI and from West Lambeth indicate that very few people had actually tried to register but been refused. In West Lambeth only 18 per cent of those who were not registered came into this category.

Respondents were then asked why they had not registered. The factor that proved to be most important for those on the streets was that they 'expected to be refused'. It seems that often people do not even try to register because the experiences of others are presented as an unbreakable rule:

No doctor in London will take you on without an address.

Single homeless people, who frequently suffer exclusion from a range of support services, often perceive health services as both unwelcoming and inaccessible.

Others pointed to their mobile way of life as a barrier to access:

I haven't registered as I don't know from one day to the next where I'm going to be.

Inflexibility of services is clearly a major issue for service providers if they are genuinely looking to improve accessibility in the future.

The majority of people who had failed to register, however, simply stated that it was 'not a priority'. It is not difficult to imagine that within an individual's hierarchy of needs the competing demands of finding a bed for the night, the next hot meal, or a source of ready cash will invariably take precedence over a medical problem. Homeless people quickly become trapped in a cycle of neglect where, as the statistics on the use of services show, preventative or primary care is missed out ensuring that most health problems have become crises by the time they are finally treated. Or as one man put it succinctly:

> I won't go to a doctor unless I'm seriously ill: and if I'm seriously ill its time to go to hospital.

There is, perhaps, another way of interpreting the low priority that many single homeless people give to registering with a GP. A final question in the West Lambeth survey asked respondents if there were any other medical services that they would like provided beyond what was already available. Although there were comparatively few responses to this open ended question it was interesting to note that by far the largest group of responses could be categorized as 'non-medical' services. This category included people who wanted more money, accommodation, information on rights or benefits, more day centres, and more recreational opportunities.

These results suggest that many single homeless people do not see medical or health services in the same terms as health professionals. Health care is perceived as being much broader than simply a series of medical interventions. In isolation, curative treatment is often seen as an irrelevance compared to the potential for effecting a meaningful change in people's health status through the improvement of material, social and environmental conditions. We will examine the implications of these interpretations for our understanding of the meaning of health towards the end of the paper.

The problem most generally cited by single homeless people who succeed in using health services, is the attitude of the health professionals that treat them. As part of a recent survey carried out in West Lambeth single homeless people were asked in what ways the existing medical services could be improved for them. After complaints about under-investment in the NHS and the waiting time for services, which we might to expect to hear from all sections of the population, complaints about the attitude of health professionals were by far the most common type of response. The strength of feeling about the perceived injustice of their treatment is clear:

> All doctors should deal with people who are homeless and take them on their lists whether they like it or not; we're just as entitled to medical treatment as anyone else.
> Doctors should have a better social understanding of people. There's only one category for people like me—dosser—and they've got no time for us.

198

We need GPs who will be sympathetic—as soon as they know you're homeless they think you're a subspecies—trash.

It would be good if they spoke to you a bit better. Their attitude to me is 'I don't want to know'. If I had money it would be different.

It should be stressed that we are not suggesting that health professionals are seen as being particularly unsympathetic or prejudicial in their treatment of homeless people, but, rather that the attitude of staff in the NHS mirrors the type of treatment that they can expect from society in general. Single homeless people have come to expect to be marginalized or excluded from almost every institution that provides support to those in need.

Barriers to providing a service as perceived by health professionals

It is recognized that many GPs feel they lack the time, resources, and information to provide an appropriate service to single homeless people. Two GP surveys conducted by FPCs in 1986 suggested that in order to enable GPs to provide a service for homeless people they required improved information about the agencies working with homeless people as well as better liaison with nursing teams and Social Services departments.

Follow-up work, however, in Bloomsbury, London, cast some doubt on the motivation of GPs to take single homeless people onto their lists in the first place (Cumming, 1986). While eleven GPs in the area had initially claimed that they were willing to take on homeless people, in practice, when presented with real patients, only three were actually prepared to do so. There are also real concerns that some of the changes proposed in the current health service reforms, such as limiting drug budgets, may act as a further disincentive to registering homeless people.

One frequently adopted solution to the problems of access facing single homeless people is the use of specialist services, that is the provision of a service exclusive to this client group. Specialist centres tend to be an *ad hoc* response offering an immediate improvement in access to care, with the long-term aim of reintegrating the users of the service into mainstream services, and thereby rendering the centres redundant.

In practice, there is little evidence that specialist services are successful at reintegrating their users into generic primary care services. The recent study of two specialist centres in London (Williams and Allen 1989) fails to throw any new light on this area. It appears that people are only reabsorbed onto general practitioners lists once they have been rehoused into permanent accommodation.

At the same time, specialist centres tend to institutionalize the discrimination and inequalities they attempt to alleviate. Once a purpose built centre is placed within an area, all other professionals seem to feel absolved of responsibility for their care. There is also some reason to doubt whether the quality of care in these parallel services is comparable to normal general practitioner surgeries. Certainly access is often limited, especially in terms of opening hours and full-time medical cover.

Can health services be changed to meet the needs of single homeless people?

The problems which single homeless people face of poor access to health services, and of the unhelpful attitudes of some health professionals, are not easily rectified in the large and often impersonal NHS. Indeed, these two problems may be seen as a reflection of a system which has become rigid and impersonal and unable to offer a caring face.

Starting from this perspective, our suggested solutions are for changes to the health care system, rather than its users, and are directed to two main areas:

1   education of health professionals;
2   current system of primary health care.

Educating health professionals

One of the recommendations in the report *From the Margins to the Mainstream* is that more information should be made available to local health professionals about the health needs of single homeless people in their area. The rationale for this recommendation was not only the apparent lack of understanding, shown by some health workers of the specific problems of access to, and use of, services which single homeless people face, but also that there was so little recording of whether service users were single homeless people. Having information about housing and family is important for planning discharge care, but more critically, because decent housing is, we would have thought, a basic prerequisite for health.

While providing practical information for health workers will help them to meet their single homeless clients' needs for food or shelter, it seems that a fundamental problem for many health workers is what they understand by health, and therefore what they understand by 'ill health' and 'improving health'.

It is uncommon, still, for medical and nursing students to spend time learning about the rather philosophical concepts of the meanings of health and illness. At Liverpool University Medical School there is a full-time lecturer in philosophy attached to the department who runs a Master's course in medical ethics (Seedhouse, 1989). But this is an exception, not a rule. Yet health workers must surely have as a goal that they are improving the health of their patients or clients; the breadth with which the term 'health' is used will certainly affect the interventions deemed appropriate by health workers, and the criteria by which they measure the effectiveness of outcomes.

Giving a meaning to health and health care

There are a number of definitions and theories of what health means, and in discussing them we have drawn heavily on the work of Seedhouse (1988).

The World Health Organization's define health as::

> a state of complete physical, mental and social wellbeing, and not merely the absence of disease.

While the aspirations of this definition are laudable, in practice it is almost impossible to use it as an achievable goal for health workers to have for the effects of their care, no matter which population is being cared for. Others have discussed the difficulties of defining wellbeing (Seedhouse 1988; Coutts and Hardy 1985). It is almost impossible to measure 'wellness', except, perhaps in objective physical terms. Our research has shown that many single homeless people do not complain about their physical health, even though, objectively, it is poorer than other population groups.

Other theories of what health is are based on social functioning. These theories contend that a person is healthy if they can perform activities expected of them. This implies that not so functioning is the opposite of health, yet there are those who wish to change their lives by not fulfilling the expectations of their social role. Such changes may be positive or negative, but do not necessarily indicate illness.

The most well known of the proponents of the social theory of health is Talcott Parsons. His critics say that his theory works to maintain society in its present state (Seedhouse 1988). Clearly such a theory is inadequate for single homeless people, who may wish to change their individual state, or for whom societal changes may be of considerable benefit.

Two other theories are related. The first is that health can somehow be 'given', rather like a commodity. This implies that people who give health care, give health. This theory is strongly related to medical practice, which aims to cure. The second, related theory is that health comes from inner strength—the indomitable human spirit. Both these theories suggest that ill health is related to failure—either that of the health worker, or of the individual. The latter is too vague to be of much practical use—how is it possible to increase a person's inner strength?

Finally, there is a theory that health is an ability to adapt. Perhaps the best known of the definitions of this theory is that one by Katherine Mansfield (1977):

> By health I mean the power to live a full, adult, living, breathing life in close contact with what I love.... I want to be all that I am capable of becoming (pp 279–279)

Other versions of this theory have been put forward by Ivan Illich, who is a radical opponent of medical science. He believes that medical science can actually cause harm by exerting professional control over an individual's natural ability to adapt to life changes. He says::

> Health designates a process of adaptation. It is not the result of instinct, but of an autonomous yet culturally shaped reaction to socially created reality. It designates the ability to adapt to changing environments, to growing up and ageing, to healing when damaged, to suffering, and to the peaceful expectation of death. Health embraces the future as well, and therefore includes anguish and the inner resources to live with it.... Health is a task, and as such is not comparable to the physiological balance of the beasts. Success in this personal task is in large part the result of self-awareness, self-discipline, and inner resources by which each person regulates his own daily rhythm and actions, his diet, and his sexual activity. (Illich 1977, pp 273–274).

Seedhouse (1988) has described this group of theories as 'sugar-coated' and vague. Certainly, it would be difficult to construct achievable goals from them. However, the theory seems to come closest to linking health to quality of life—implying the achievement of personal potential and a comfortable balance. As with other theories described here, there is a danger (with this one) that it could result in 'blaming' an unhealthy person for their unhealthiness. If a person is unable to adapt to changes then is that due to their own personal inadequacy?

It has been important to consider these definitions of health in relation to working with single homeless people. It could be easy to think that the purpose of a project to improve health care for a group of often physically unfit people is to improve their physical health. This would severely limit the effect of the project and would have disappointing results. How effective can treatment be for disease if poor social conditions remain unchanged? On the other hand, by adopting a broader, more philosophical definition of health, it is harder to define achievable aims for health work, and easier to blame individuals for their own ill health.

The definition of health which seems to meet our need for a comprehensive achievable aim is that developed by Seedhouse (1988). He concludes that health is a foundation from which chosen goals can be achieved. To achieve these goals it may be necessary to remove obstacles, and that work for health can involve helping clients to identify and remove obstacles.

Seedhouse argues that there are certain central conditions for health, and that these should be primary concerns for health workers. These are:

1 Basic needs of food, drink, shelter, warmth and purpose in life.
2 Access to the widest possible information about all factors which have an influence on a person's life.
3 Skill and confidence to assimilate this information.....
4 ....Recognition that.... people are complex wholes who cannot be fully understood separated from the influence of their environment, which is itself a whole of which they are a part..... The recognition that a person should not strive to fulfil personal potentials which will undermine the basic foundations for achievement of other people (pp 61–62)

By viewing central conditions for health in this broad way, it becomes clear that to work for health demands a commitment to social and economic change, and education, as well as to individual physical health.

The relevance of this model of health for work with people who are often deprived of warmth, privacy, close relationships and shelter, is, in part, obvious. Health interventions cannot ignore such deprivation, and should seek ways to facilitate change.

There are dangers in this model, the chief of which is that it could result in individuals being blamed for their own inadequacies eg not having a purpose in life, and therefore not becoming a 'successful' citizen. However, the other way of looking at the model makes it revolutionary in that much economic policy and many social systems must change if everyone who is single and homeless is to have their basic needs met.

Re-examining primary health care—a model for change

The Declaration of Alma-Ata in 1978 specified the essential principle of primary health care as:

Accessibility to all populations.

Maximum individual and community involvement in service planning and operation.

Emphasis on care which is preventive and promotive, rather than curative.

Use of appropriate and acceptable technology.

Integration of health development with comprehensive social and economic development.

Primary health care is not usually related to these principles in this country, largely because, we contend, they are thought to be more suitable for developing communities rather than our wealthy western society. Yet if we are to face the inequalities which exist in our society and which most certainly influence health (Whitehead 1987), then to be effective, primary health care must surely espouse these principles.

In line with this concept of primary care we are looking to develop a new form of access to services which is not simply accessible first aid but first contact care that is appropriate to users. It is also important to develop a model that addresses the current inequalities in access without creating parallel 'ghetto' clinics.

A useful model can be found in the Province of Quebec in Canada where a network of Local Community Health Clinics (known as CLSC—the initials of the French translation) have been developed. They were started in order to supplement the general practice system, providing a combination of health and social care free to a local population in places where services are not easily accessible, such as rural and inner city areas. CLSC clinics have a wide range of staff, including nurse practitioners and other nurses, doctors, social workers, counsellors, health educationalists, dietitians and dentists. They have also succeeded in being highly accessible in a number of ways. One particular CLSC is situated in a metro station in Montreal, which is widely used by the population passing through the station. It offers a high standard of care and surroundings to all. A number of CLSCs are open long hours to meet the needs of the population likely to use it. There is also a strong emphasis on the importance of friendly reception staff and welcoming waiting areas.

The feasibility of a similar style of walk-in clinic, situated near, or in, Waterloo Station in central London, is currently being investigated. It is envisaged that the new centre would meet the needs of anyone passing through the area, including commuters or tourists using the station, but that it would also offer a new, immediate form of access to services for those who had previously found themselves excluded. It is expected that the new health facilities would offer a wide range of individual consultation services with many professional groups. It is also hoped that the clinic could offer groupwork and support in various aspects of lifestyle, such as relaxation, stopping smoking, healthier diets, or coping with stress. The new centre could provide useful insights into why some people do not fully use existing general practitioner services. There is also considerable scope for a centre of this kind to relieve the local accident and emergency department of some of the 'inappropriate' attenders, presenting with primary care needs, who make up a large part of their current workload. Recognizing that such a health centre might cause antagonism from other near-by general practitioner services, their views on the scheme would be sought. It is hoped that local GPs would be able to work at the health centre on a sessional basis, and therefore feel it to be a cooperative, rather than competitive venture. Training and support would also be given to all staff to ensure a high standard of communication skills, a thorough understanding of the needs of different population groups and ways of meeting those needs.

It is important to remember, however, that the most pressing need of those who are homeless is for a home. Innovations in accessing health care will not in themselves lead to a real improvement in health. Such changes are irrelevant if they are not accompanied by a genuine improvement in the material and environmental conditions experienced by homeless people.

References

Bone M 1984 *Registration with General Medical Practitioners in inner London: a survey carried out on* behalf of the DHSS. HMSO, London

Coutts L C and Hardy L K 1985. *Teaching for health.* Churchill Livingstone, Edinburgh

Cumming J 1986 *No room for health? health care services for the hostel homeless in Bloomsbury.* London School of Hygiene and Tropical Medicine, London

Illich I 1977 *Limits to Medicine.* Penguin books, Harmondsworth

Mansfield K 1977 *Letters and journals.* Penguin books, Harmondsworth

OPCS 1986 *General household survey.* HMSO, London

Seedhouse D 1988 *Health: the foundations for achievement.* John Wiley, Chichester

Stern R and Stilwell B 1989. *From the Margins to the Mainstream: Collaboration in planning services with single homeless people.* West Lambeth Health Authority, London

Whitehead M 1987 *The health divide: Inequalities in health in the 1980's.* Health Education Council, London

Williams S and Allen I 1989 *Health Care for single homeless people.* Policy Studies Institute, London

14 Health care for single homeless people

Sandra Williams and Isobel Allen

The Department of Health has for some time been concerned about the delivery of primary health care services to homeless people and has encouraged the efforts made by some family practitioner committees (FPCs) and GPs to find locally acceptable solutions to the problem. In 1985 the Department decided to establish two pilot schemes for providing health care to homeless people in Inner London so that the issues could be examined in more detail. The schemes were funded to run provisionally for three years and a major departure from the way in which general practice is organized was that they were staffed with salaried doctors.

The Policy Studies Institute was asked to evaluate both projects and we found them to have made a valuable contribution to the debate about the best way of helping people who are often thought to be on the fringes of society. In conducting our evaluation of the schemes we inevitably examined and highlighted many of the key issues relating to the provision of primary health care for homeless people more generally. This paper describes the design and method of the research and discusses the findings and recommendations that ensued.

Background to the evaluation

The pilot schemes were set up by the Department of Health and Social Security (DHSS) in 1986 to provide primary health care to homeless people. The schemes were based in two units, one in Camden and one in Tower Hamlets, administered respectively by the Camden and Islington and the City and East London FPCs. Each unit was staffed by a multidisciplinary team. The team in Camden comprised a salaried doctor, a nurse, and a project administrator. In Tower Hamlets the team included a salaried doctor, a community psychiatric nurse (who left shortly after the project started), an alcohol counsellor, a social worker, and a project administrator. Each unit had its own premises but was not generally available for consultation there. Instead, team members provided their services on an outreach basis, visiting a number of day centres, night shelters and hostels where the homeless people were known to congregate.

During the monitoring period, which was the calender year of 1987, the project doctor in East London held regular clinics in five centres; these included two day centres, an evening centre, a short-stay hostel and a detoxification unit. In the same period the doctor in Camden established regular clinics in two day centres and one night shelter.

The objectives of the pilot schemes were to identify and contact as many homeless people as practicable within the locality of the FPCs, gain their confidence, diagnose and treat their morbidity and, wherever possible, secure their admission to the list of a general medical practitioner. The main aim of the evaluation was to test the objectives of the schemes. The Department envisaged that essentially this would be a descriptive study, looking at the organization and functioning of the two health care teams; the referral patterns into and out of the schemes; and the incidence of morbidity and mortality of the consumers. The Department also hoped that it would assess the views both of professionals and voluntary workers, as well as clients themselves, on the delivery of primary care to the homeless. It was hoped that we might develop measures of outcome to test the effectiveness of the schemes on the health and wellbeing of the consumers—the homeless people.

Project design

We based our study on two main methods of research: (i) a system for monitoring the take-up of services in both project areas; and (ii) in-depth personal interviews.

Monitoring use and users

We developed a system of monitoring the activity, organization, referral patterns and functioning of the pilot health care teams, using information from the medical record system operated by both pilot teams. We wanted to provide a description of the day-

207

to-day work of the two schemes and we also wanted to give detailed information about the users of the schemes. This included: numbers; age and sex of clients; sources of referral into the scheme; whether or not users were registered with a GP; what use clients made of the services; the kind of problems with which they presented themselves; referrals out of the scheme; and outcome, as far as it was known, both in terms of the individual's health and wellbeing and in terms of service provision and take-up.

In developing this monitoring system we worked closely with both teams to establish a medical record system which could be used by them for practical purposes and by us for our research and monitoring purposes. Devising and setting up a medical record system which would satisfy our needs for the evaluation and which was also acceptable to service providers in both project sites was not easy. There were differences of opinion between the researchers and the teams (and also within the teams) about the *amount* and *kind* of information it was feasible and acceptable to ask the doctors and other team members to record. Information that would have been useful to the evaluation was not necessarily seen by team members as relevant to providing care.

We negotiated with team members for three months before arriving at agreed formats for the medical record card and the contact sheets which were used by both teams. The *medical record card* indicated the person's registration number, recorded brief personal details, and was used by the team for recording notes relating to each consultation. The medical record cards provided us with a record of the total number of different *individuals* seen by each project team during the calendar year of 1987. Team members also recorded information about each consultation they had with a user on a *contact sheet* and this information in a coded form provided us with a database of information about the total number of *consultations* made by homeless people with project team members during the twelve month monitoring period. We used patient registration numbers to identify individuals: patients' names were not used by the research team.

To give some idea of the size of the database generated by the medical record cards and contact sheets, in east London a total of 885 individuals used the pilot scheme one or more times during the calendar year of 1987.

These 885 individuals made a total of 3,198 consultations during this period. In Camden a total of 576 individuals used the pilot scheme in that area one or more times during the twelve month monitoring period and between them made a total of 2,022 consultations. These figures are not comparable because the size and composition of the teams were different.

In-depth personal interviews

We wanted to establish what everyone concerned felt about the schemes, and how they perceived them to be working. We were convinced that before any assessment could be made of the relative success or failure, or strengths or weaknesses of the schemes, it was vital to know what the providers and the consumers thought about them. We also thought that it was important to seek the views of professionals and voluntary workers involved in the provision of health care and social care to homeless people. Therefore, we designed the study to include personal interviews with:

1 Samples of clients or consumers of the services offered by the two pilot health care teams. Interviews were achieved with 190 homeless people, 50 per cent of whom had used the schemes' services.
2 All members of the health care teams and their managers.
3 Samples of professionals concerned with the statutory provision of health or social services in the localities of the pilot projects. We interviewed 76 professionals providing care in the community and fifteen professionals either working in or taking referrals from the accident and emergency departments of two large London teaching hospitals—one in east London and one in west London.
4 Representatives and workers from fourteen local voluntary agencies offering health care, counselling or social services to homeless people.
5 Wardens of the day centres, night shelters and hostels where the project doctors had established regular clinics.

These interviews were conducted during the twelve month monitoring period. They provided an immense amount of data about health care for homeless people from a number of different perspectives. In particular, we broke new ground in the debate about health care for the homeless in that we introduced the voice of the consumer. We talked to homeless people themselves about their health care experiences. We accepted that there were many problems involved in the measurement and use of consumer opinion, but we were convinced that the story needed to be told from the consumer's point of view and that their perceptions of the pilot schemes were an essential component of the evaluation.

Not everyone agreed with us. Project team members, particularly the doctors, were unhappy about us talking to the users of their services, that is, the homeless people. They raised doubts about the usefulness of client evaluation and emphasised the problem of reliability. More importantly for them, they were worried that our talking to clients would affect the service they provided. They thought that if people associated being interviewed with using the service, they would stop using it. These views had major implications for our proposed client evaluation. We had to ensure, so far as was possible, that our interviews with clients were detached in time from their consultation with the project doctor. In practice this meant that we could not interview homeless people at any of the centres when a project doctor was holding a surgery there.

In the event we interviewed a total of 190 homeless people, of whom 50 per cent had used the schemes' services and 50 per cent had not; 90 of the interviews were in East London and 100 interviews in Camden. They took place in day centres, night shelters or hostels in both areas where regular clinics had been set up by the project doctors. These interviews were done on a quota sampling basis because it was impossible to find a suitable sampling frame which would have enabled us to select a random sample of interviewees. So that we could explore possible seasonable variations in service take-up or problems presented, half the interviews were conducted in June 1987 and the other half were conducted in November 1987.

Although the sites for the interviews and the quota controls were determined in advance, the final selection of people for interview was left to the interviewers, who were carefully briefed about contact and interview procedure. This briefing, however, could not completely prepare them for the culture shock they experienced on their first visit to a centre. One of the interviewers vividly captured her reaction:

> From the moment of leaving the Tube there seemed to be nothing but shuffling old men in grey overcoats moving slowly towards the crypt. Just total culture shock—so many, it seemed, in such a small area accentuated by the low ceilings. It seemed like stepping back into something medieval.

Surprisingly few people refused to be interviewed—of those approached only 19 per cent refused. The topics we talked to homeless people about included: their attitudes towards the services provided by the pilot schemes; what they liked or disliked about the way the services were organized and delivered; how they thought these services compared with other sources of health care; the extent to which they wanted to be on a GP's list or whether they preferred to use the special service. In our main report on the evaluation (Williams and Allen 1989) we make extensive use of verbatim quotes from respondents to illustrate points made. Much of the richness and poignancy of the data we collected would have been lost if we had not presented their views in their own words. It was often difficult to get them to focus on the questions. Instead of framing specific answers to questions, they often related snippets of their life story to illustrate their views or their experiences of health care. Some of these stories were compelling to listen to but they were time consuming. This has a bearing on their use of health care services because if they had difficulty in concentrating on direct questions posed by the interviewer, it is probable that they may have problems in an ordinary GP's surgery where the doctor may not have the time or inclination to listen.

We interviewed project team members at three points during the monitoring period in order to record any changes or developments, either in the structure and functioning of the pilot scheme, or in their own views and understanding of the scheme. We also conducted in-depth interviews with the chairmen and administrators of the two managing FPCs. From both service providers and managers we wanted to know their assessment of the impact of the scheme and, looking to the future, whether they thought that some form of special separate provision should continue after the initial funding for the project expired. The changes in team personnel had implications for the evaluation as well as for the service provided under the scheme. The membership of the team we interviewed at the end of the monitoring period was substantially different from that at the outset. Indeed, in the east London project there had been a complete change of staff by the end of the twelve months.

We also interviewed the wardens in the centres where the project doctors had established regular clinics, both at the beginning of 1987 and at the end of the year. These interviews provided a valuable insight into the health problems and experiences of those people who attended the centres. They also highlighted some of the wardens' major concerns; for example, the extent of mental health problems among their clients and the lack of resources to deal with these problems; the extent of alcohol abuse and the lack of detoxification facilities.

How appropriate are mainstream primary health care services to the needs and circumstances of homeless people? Do health care professionals who provide these services think that homeless people can be integrated into mainstream provision or do they favour special provision of primary care services for the single homeless? How far do their views coincide or conflict with the views of those working in the voluntary sector who have an interest in the health care of homeless people?

To explore these and related issues we interviewed a total of 105 health and social service professionals working in the localities of the two pilot schemes. We also covered the same ground in interviews with fourteen representatives of local organizations concerned with the health and housing needs of homeless people. Our sample of health and social service professionals included GPs, district nurses, community psychiatric nurses, local authority social workers, and hospital accident and emergency staff. One of the most revealing comments about the consequences of living rough or in squalid conditions was made by one of the social workers in the sample. She said 'When you talk to someone who seems chronologically ten years older than they are you get some idea of the wear and tear on the body'.

Problems and issues

Before discussing our findings and recommendations it is helpful to be aware of some of the problems and issues we encountered in undertaking this piece of evaluative research and which had an impact on the conduct of the research. Not all the problems we experienced stemmed from the fact that this was an evaluation study. Some of the problems arose simply because the homeless population was difficult to survey.

Method

When this study was being set up we were involved in a methodological debate about how the evaluation should proceed. There was a clear division between two groups: clinicians, who wanted us to set up a medical model at the outset and to devise clear outcome measures before data was collected; and social scientists who favoured a more flexible framework for evaluative research, which acknowledged that initiatives often change in midstream. The scope of evaluative research was a key issue; whether the aim should be to assess the extent to which the original aim is being, or has been, realised; or whether, in order to learn lessons from the experience which is being evaluated, the aim should be to look at objectives, inputs, the process of implementation and the measurement of outcomes as part of that whole experience. In this study we took the latter approach.

Outcome measures

The Department hoped that we would be able to develop measures of outcome to test the effectiveness of the schemes on the health and well being of homeless people. In trying to develop these outcome measures we were confronted not only by the well documented difficulties associated with assessing outcomes in general practice, but also the problem that the population we were surveying was not stable and was virtually impossible to follow-up. It was difficult to measure the extent to which the long term aim of securing the admission of as many homeless people as possible to the list of a GP had been achieved. Several factors contributed to the problem. In particular, the currency of registration for homeless people was usually temporary registration, not permanent registration. Moreover, medical confidentiality restricted access to information provided for registration purposes. Realistically we were only able to look at outcomes in terms of 'terminating actions' to consultations individuals had with project team members.

Professional autonomy

We had to overcome the initial problem that team members felt threatened by an external evaluation and were defensive. The doctors in particular were unhappy about being evaluated by non-clinicians. There was some confusion on their part as to whether we were primarily evaluating the individuals providing the service, the quality of the service provided, or the pilot schemes as a method of delivering primary health care to homeless people. These aspects are difficult to separate but our emphasis was on the problem of providing health care to homeless people and this problem was precisely one of the organization and functioning of the services themselves.

Findings from the study

In discussing the main findings and recommendations of the study, we examined four main areas.

1 How did the pilot schemes work and what actually happened?
2 What were the problems and difficulties encountered both by the teams and the researchers?
3 What did they achieve?
4 What did we recommend and why?

Services provided and use of the schemes

In both areas, a small multidisciplinary team of professionals visited a limited number of day centres, night shelters and hostels and provided primary health care to homeless people who attended those centres. They did not provide any service outside these centres and they did not provide any services outside office hours. Each team employed a salaried doctor rather than using local GPs. The people they saw could not register with them, as they did not provide 24-hour cover and visited each centre once, twice or at most three times a week.

The Camden team was very small, with just a doctor and a nurse. The nurse undertook some health promotion work in add–ition to general nursing duties. The City and East London team included an alcohol counsellor and social worker as well as the doctor, and during the monitoring period it had a community psy-chiatric nurse for the first three months.

It should be stressed that in both areas there was an additional nurse who was not officially part of the team, but in fact worked so closely with the team members that it was difficult to separate her contributions from the work of the team. In East London the nurse was employed by the health authority and in Camden by the West London Day Centre. Around a quarter of all consultations with the two teams were made with these nurses, and any assess-ment of the figures must take this into consideration.

Who used the services? The overwhelming majority of users were male, white, unemployed, single—or living as single—and were mainly homeless, although quite a few were living in long-stay hostels and as many as a quarter of those we interviewed said they had their own accommodation. The people who used the services were people who attended the centres in which they were provid-ed. This meant that the services did not reach many homeless women and people from ethnic minorities who were unlikely to use this kind of street agency, and, although there had been hopes of developing outreach work, the services did not reach homeless families at all.

Why did people use the services and what kind of help were they seeking? They did not necessarily use them for general medi-cal services. Although many people consulted the doctor for respi-ratory or skin problems or for help with injuries or wounds, a high proportion of patients were said to have mental health problems and many of the consultations were for alcohol related problems. (Details of the consultations are given in the main report on the study, see Williams and Allen, 1989). It should be noted that only just over half the consultations in both areas were with the doc-tors. The nurses saw a lot of people, and many of these consulta-tions were for advice or help about social or medical problems rather than for actual treatment. Some people clearly just wanted a chat with someone who was helpful, friendly and kind, and users often commented on how much they liked the service because team members treated them like human beings— something they often appeared to find in short supply in other areas of their lives.

We found that more people using the services said they were registered with a doctor than is generally assumed—nearly half the users of the East London scheme and over a third of the Camden users. Among those we interviewed, who included users and non-users of the services, the proportion saying they were registered was higher. But, of course, registration with a doctor may be a bit academic if your doctor is in Scotland and you are in London. Nevertheless, we found that even if people were registered they might well use the schemes' services simply because they were there, close at hand, staffed by friendly people with time to sit and chat and explain things, and available without the hassle of getting past the GP's receptionist, braving the waiting room and seeing a doctor who might not be tuned into the rather special needs of some homeless people. Many of the people we interviewed were not people who led tidy lives which easily lent themselves to making and keeping appointments or waiting to be seen in an orderly manner.

We also found that single homeless people were not actually clamouring to register with GPs. Like many people who are housed, registering with a doctor was not a priority—they only wanted one when they were ill or in need of medical care. Many of them led rather mobile lives and if they did not know where they were likely to be next week or next month, they saw little point in plugging into a system in which many of them had little faith in any case.

We found that many of those interviewed had had fairly unhappy experiences to report about the level and type of health care they had received in the past, although we must stress that there were also reports of very good support and stable relationships with health care professionals. General practitioners themselves were not too keen on extending their services to too many single homeless people and although quite a few were happy to consider them on an individual basis, we still found that the majority interviewed held pretty stereotyped views of homeless people as being potentially dirty, drunk, and disruptive and were concerned about creating an additional burden on their workload as well as upsetting other patients in their waiting rooms. They were more likely to treat homeless people as temporary residents than to give them permanent registration, and it was clear that some used the lack of a permanent address as an excuse for not offering permanent registration.

Problems and difficulties

The problems and difficulties we encountered can be summarised under two headings—those associated with the nature and organization of the pilot schemes themselves and those associated with evaluating and assessing the success of the schemes. In fact, they had a bearing on each other, but it is useful to outline briefly the component parts of each before bringing them together.

The schemes were set up as pilots by a Government initiative, but started in rather different ways and at different times. One was grafted onto a service which was already up and running with a doctor providing sessions in certain centres, while the other was set up from scratch. Neither scheme was operating in a vacuum and there were undoubtedly a number of problems associated with territorial rights and disputes with professionals, voluntary organizations, and others working with homeless people, some of whom had understandable suspicions of new teams with no apparent track record, who had central government funding and backing and had been set up as 'model' or 'demonstration' projects.

They were set up as multidisciplinary teams, but the various members of the teams were employed by different authorities or agencies, had different lines of accountability, and had no clearly defined set of roles and responsibilities. There were problems associated with the actual management of the teams themselves, and there were definite problems at the beginning in solving apparently simple administrative matters, like how to get supplies.

The monitoring and evaluation covered a short time period, and the schemes' funding from the Department only covered a slightly longer period. There can be no doubt that many problems flowed directly from the fact that they were a group of people struggling to set up a new service with a new team while under close scrutiny and working to a tight time scale. They were under tremendous pressure to succeed—to demonstrate something—and it is hardly surprising that there were tensions and difficulties.

In the report we discuss the very important question of the problems of evaluating 'innovations', and we draw attention to the fact that the most successful innovations may rely almost exclusively on the personality and drive of an individual or group who have a 'mission' to succeed. It is not surprising that such schemes are difficult to replicate and that when the pioneer has departed, the scheme itself may lost its momentum. These pilot schemes were rather different from innovations of that kind. Much can be learnt from their experience, but they also demonstrate how difficult it is to draw up a 'model' for others from centrally 'imposed' schemes which do not spring from local initiatives and can be rather artificial.

Another of the difficulties surrounded the fact that the twin objectives—to provide a good primary health care service and to get people to register with GPs—were felt to be almost mutually exclusive by the team members, especially the doctors, who thought they could be interpreted as putting across 'mixed messages' to the users of the services.

This linked into another major difficulty which bridged the service delivery and the research and evaluation. What criteria were to be used for judging the success or lack of success of the service? It could be judged successful in getting lots of people to register with local GPs but could have failed in the objective of supplying people with a good level of service. Or it could provide such a good level of service that nobody would want to register with local GPs, or might feel rejected if the team doctors suggested they did.

What other criteria could be used? We could use the simple measure of the numbers seen. But this is a very blunt instrument, and needs to be interpreted with caution. We have no idea of the size of the potential demand. The take-up figures might reflect only a fraction of what is needed or might reflect over provision. And again, high numbers of repeat visits might indicate 'failure' in getting people to register with GPs. We could not really look at outcomes, in the conventional sense. Outcome measurement is difficult enough in general practice in any case, but with this client group it was even more difficult in that they were not a stable population, doctors had difficulty in obtaining reliable medical histories, and they were often impossible to follow-up.

Essentially, a variety of measures was required, including those based on the views of the users, the other professionals and voluntary agencies in the area, and the wardens of the centres where the teams worked. These are important indicators of how the services were seen, known about, and accepted.

Achievements

The users liked the services on the whole. They liked the people providing them, they liked being able to use a service which was available where they were, at a time convenient to them, staffed by friendly, kind and accepting people who did not adopt judgemental attitudes and were prepared to give them time and chat to them. But there was evidence that many of the consultations were not strictly for general medical care. What was demonstrated was a need for more counselling, advice, and nursing care rather than general medical care on the one hand, and on the other hand there was a very clear need for more specialist services for mental health and alcohol related problems.

The wardens of the centres were particularly appreciative of the teams. They provided them with specialist back-up and support, particularly in dealing with clients with mental health and alcohol related problems. One of the most useful outcomes was the training element provided by the alcohol counsellor to staff dealing with alcohol problems on a day-to-day basis. Other professionals and voluntary agencies were less positive about the efforts of the teams. There was considerable evidence that many knew nothing about the existence of the schemes, and this was perhaps particularly worrying among the doctors working in the accident and emergency departments of local hospitals, who saw so many people who could well have benefited from the teams' services.

Neither project had made much progress in getting people registered with local GPs. Given the ambivalence the project doctors felt about such a recommendation, this was perhaps not surprising, but the question remains of how far such an objective was achievable in any case. There was a general consensus among professionals and others that although there were many who could be encouraged to register there would always be some who would never be willing or able to do so, and there would always be others who would never be accepted, however hard everyone tried.

Recommendations

In spite of the achievements of the teams, we did not recommend their continuation in the form in which they had been working. We recommended that health care services for single homeless people should be firmly rooted within mainstream services, and that the aim should be for GPs to provide general medical services for them within their own surgeries or in special sessions or clinics which should be set up in day centres, night shelters or hostels. We recommended that consideration would have to be given to how these practitioners should be paid for providing these services outside their own surgeries. We felt that any advantages in using salaried doctors for providing special health care services of this kind were far outweighed by the disadvantages. In general, we thought there should be more education and discussion with GPs on the special needs and problems of single homeless people, and we recommended that FPCs should take a more proactive role in encouraging a change in attitudes towards homeless people among GPs.

We felt there was a danger in providing special services to homeless people through special teams it may serve to marginalize people who were already operating on the fringes of society. We saw no reason why services recognizing the special needs of single homeless people could not be provided within the mainstream services. However, we did recognize that there was a need for special services within these mainstream services, particularly in connection with mental health and alcohol related problems. The wardens, who were in constant contact with the men using the centres pointed out the desperate need for more detoxification units and for much more help with alcohol counselling and mental health problems. As we look at the increasing numbers of former residents of our psychiatric hospitals roaming the streets of our big cities, it is difficult not to agree with the wardens.

The pilot schemes certainly underlined the need for a multidisciplinary approach to the delivery of health care to single homeless people. The importance of the services offered by the nurses, the alcohol counsellor and the social worker was recognized and appreciated by the users of the service and some of the professionals. We recommended that much more health promotion and health education should be made available for single homeless people, and the multidisciplinary approach offered ways of achieving this.

Finally, we stressed throughout the report that single homeless people do not constitute a homogeneous group of people for whom one type of health care can be prescribed. We need a number of different approaches to deliver health care to people who certainly require it but have different needs. There is no one easy solution.

References

Williams S, Allen I 1989 *Health care for single homeless people*. Policy Studies Institute, London

15 Towards 2000

Susan J Smith
Ann McGuckin and
Robin Knill-Jones

In Britain, the 1980s and 1990s can be best described as a period
of welfare restructuring (Smith 1989a). Across the full range of
public services we have seen a radical renegotiation of the social
contract, introducing changes unparalleled since the setting up of
the postwar welfare state. This restructuring is not a simple product
of adjustment to the dynamics of supply and demand for public services and social welfare. Rather, it is a product of the political management of a set of complex economic changes.

These economic changes can be thought of in global terms as
part of a process most often described as a transition from organized to disorganized capitalism, from Fordism to flexible accumulation, or, more broadly, from modernism to postmodernism (this
transition is discussed at length by a variety of authors, but it it
most helpfully summarized by Albertsen 1988, Harvey 1989,
Lash and Urry 1987). The significance of these shifts for the
British welfare state is that they represent a step towards the
internationalization of capital, labour and finance markets. They
testify to a process of global economic integration which means
that states have less scope to protect their economies from com-
petition in world markets, and that politicians may be less able or
willing to use taxation policies as a resource for offsetting economic inequalities through welfare transfers.

As Jessop (1988) points out, there are in principle a variety of
political options available to governments for managing these far-
reaching economic changes. In the context of British neoconser-
vatism, however, some strategies have proved more viable than
others: notably, the majority of politically acceptable options centre on changing the social role of the state in order to reduce public expenditure and free up the market. The role of both central
and local government is therefore viewed less as one concerned

with providing goods and services along redistributive lines and more as a means of bolstering the market and meeting the needs of the private sector. The thrust of welfare restructuring has therefore been away from subsidies for collective consumption, and away from policies associated with the redistribution of wealth. The trend is, instead towards more selective social policies which draw new boundaries between the 'deserving' and 'undeserving' poor and are linked to expenditure regimes designed primarily to support market principles (Kearns and Smith 1990).

It is important to recognise that this neoliberal strategy is not the only route available to governments which seek to renegotiate the boundaries between civil society and the state during a period of global economic upheaval (Keane 1988). However, given the political realities of (post) modern Britain, this setting must be our starting point. It is a setting which forces us to reassess the rights (as well as the social obligations) of people with medical needs. It leads us to question the extent to which housing for health is to be viewed as a market strategy and the extent to which it is to be part of the package of citizenship entitlements which the state guarantees. It raises, too, the question of whether and to what extent these two elements of health care servicing—via the state and via the market—are compatible. We address this question by considering, in turn, the restructuring of the housing system, the reorganization of the National Health Service and the reorientation of community care.

Renegotiating the social contract

Housing

Housing has been at the leading edge of welfare restructuring in the last 15 years (Forrest and Murie 1989; Clapham et al 1990). It is the first major public service in which a shift from the state to the market was associated with substantial cutbacks in public expenditure. Thus although all governments have favoured the extension of owner-occupation throughout the second half of the twentieth century, the *1980 Housing Act* was a landmark in giving council tenants, for the first time, the *right* to buy their home (and encouraging them to do so with substantial discounts and favourable mortgage terms). During the 1980s, therefore, the council rented sector shrank not only proportionately (relative to owner-occupation) but also in absolute terms.

On the one hand, the policies which underpin the privatization of public housing can be seen as a means of extending a fundamental economic right to participate in the market place to a wider proportion of the population. Indeed, from a neoliberal perspective, this ability to compete in the economy is the key to mobilizing all other fundamental citizenship entitlements. Although the notion of a property owning democracy is partly political rhetoric, it is also an acknowledgement that it is better, in a society where most of the national wealth is privatized, for property ownership to be concentrated into the hands of a large rather than smaller proportion of the population. The extension of home ownership has, moreover, benefited many people, providing them with an environment in which they feel safe, secure and in control, as well as with a (usually) appreciating capital asset and a potentially cheap source of housing services in old age. In all these respects home ownership can be beneficial to people with medical needs in the same way as it can benefit those in good health—even though it is likely that people with health problems have less access to this sector overall.

On the other hand, the extension of home ownership has gone on alongside the 'residualization' of public renting. There is some debate over the meaning of this term, but most authors use it to refer to the selective shrinking of the council stock together with the changing character of council tenants. Malpass and Murie (1982 p.174) define it as a process whereby 'public housing moves towards a position in which it provides only a 'safety net' for those who for reasons of poverty, age or infirmity cannot obtain suitable accommodation in the private sector', The public sector is effectively becoming the welfare arm of the housing system just at the time when the overall quality, desirability and indeed 'healthiness' of the stock that remains is being called into question. By the mid-1980s, the Audit Commission (1986) had discovered that some 85 per cent of council owned dwellings required repairs and improvements at a total cost of around £20 billion. For whatever reason, it is increasingly clear that policies towards council renting are creating an inferior tenure sector. This means—even in neoliberal terms—that sick people forced to rely on public housing are losing out in terms of their entitlement to a decent home; and those who currently own, but might choose to rent if suitable accommodation were available, are effectively constrained in their tenure choice.

The housing association sector has become the main alternative to council housing for people who require caring services and who wish to rent at subsidized rates. This sector accounts for a small but growing proportion of the total housing stock. However, the passage of the *1988 Housing Act* significantly changed its role. Housing associations were grouped with private landlords as part of the independent rented sector. The clear aim here is to move housing associations to a more market-orientated world, and this has implications for who secures a tenancy and for who is represented on management committees (Kearns 1990). This new market orientation could compromize the role of the housing associations as the spearhead of the 'special needs' movement, and it could undermine that sector's attempts to provide decent affordable homes for people with health problems.

The thrust of the major Housing Acts of the 1980s is, in short, towards a more market-orientated housing system. But even a cursory review of the major trends indicates that this may not be a more healthy housing system. The thrust of housing policy may, moreover, limit rather than extend the housing options available to people with medical needs. These limitations may be doubly problematic if taken in conjunction with changes in the organization (and perhaps availability) of the NHS.

Health

In the last five years, the NHS has been subject to as much, if not more, scrutiny as the public sectors of the housing system. The white paper *Working for Patients* (Secretaries of State for Health, Wales, Northern Ireland, Scotland 1989a) which was published in January 1989 may, indeed, signal the most significant changes to the NHS since its inception in 1948. Like the Audit Commission's (1986a) report on housing management in the public sector, the white paper aims to tackle what it sees as a problem not of the overall amount of resources earmarked for the NHS but rather as a problem of the way these resources are used. The white paper therefore aims to create an internal or private market within the NHS which will be arbitrated by managers not clinicians. The two most controversial elements of this package have proved to be the decision to create self-governing hospital trusts and the attempt to assign practice budgets to general practitioners (Beck and Adam 1990).

Some of these changes clearly have a bearing on the project of housing for health. They do not mean that the majority of health care will cease to be free at the point of consumption. The NHS is not being privatized in the same way as the housing system, though there is little doubt that the changes will open up new possibilities for private sector involvement (Glennerster et al 1990). Nevertheless, clients' ability to pay should not be a criterion used by clinicians when deciding who to treat and by what remedy. On the other hand, financial considerations will intrude into health care decisions more than they have in the past. Budget holding GPs, for instance, may be tempted to choose treatments on financial rather than clinical grounds (Bury 1990), and it is a short step from this to selecting patients according to the same criteria (for example by preferentially accepting those who cost less and who will comply with practice targets by turning up for screening programmes, immunizations and so on). This means that homeless people may continue to lose out in terms of access to health care; and it may mean that people living in the worst housing environments also receive less rather than more services (despite the introduction of deprivation payments in April 1990 to allow for the high workloads and pressure on GPs in the most underprivileged regions). Examining some of the key trends here, Paton (1989) fears that:'There is likely to be a flight of provision from poor areas, with residual populations suffering as their institutions or GP practices become more run-down, with less subscriptions and less financing' (p 138). At best, there seems to be a danger that budget holding practices which are 'testing the market' may do so to the detriment of overall health care planning for their district (Ford 1990).

There is, however, a more fundamental undercurrent to the 1989 white paper, and that is the shift towards a 'mixed economy of care'. This refers to the enticing notion that is is acceptable, even desirable, to use a variety of market and state strategies to deliver health services providing that such services reach those who need them in adequate amounts. This notion of welfare pluralism is increasingly of interest to analysts of social policy (Clapham et al 1990; Deakin 1987). The problem with this kind of thinking in the health care field is that we know that markets cannot be relied on to secure particular sets of resources to particular individuals: even the proponents of the marketplace (Friedman and Hayek included) are agreed on that fact. The point here is that if, among the suite of entitlements citizens receive in return for paying their taxes and obeying the law, there lurks a right to health care (and this has certainly been the case in British health policy for the last half century): then the introduction of a market model is almost certain to begin to compromise this right. As Raymond Plant (1989) observes in his powerful defence of just this right: 'given that markets cannot of themselves secure rights... and given that there is a defensible case for claiming such a right, then the role of markets and privatization in health care must be limited' (p 16). The thrust of the argument of most contributors to this book is that the effective right to health care needs to be extended rather than restricted, and that those whose rights are most difficult to mobilize are often those least able to compete in the market place. Therefore, notwithstanding the many beneficial changes that the white paper promises (Community Health Resource Unit 1990), it is important not to ignore the challenge that it deflects attention away from the underfunding of the NHS (hitherto the guarantor of the public's entitlement to medical care). It is hard, too, to ignore the challenge that many of these changes will introduce to the UK many of the problems associated with health care servicing which already being experienced in the USA, without significantly benefiting those whose health needs are most pressing (Paton 1990).

Community care

The link between a restructured housing system and a reorganised national health service hinges on the concept of community care, which mediates between where people live and the type and quality of services they receive. The idea of community care has a long history in this country: governments were committed to the concept by the *National Assistance Act of 1948*, and it has always been recognized as a key to success of the process of deinstitutionalization. That it has signally failed in this role can scarcely be questioned (O'Donnell 1989; Weller 1986), and most commentators welcomed the Government's review of community care following the Audit Commission's (1986b) complaints about its fragmentary nature and poor coordination. As a consequence of this review, community care has become the third health related policy arena to undergo a radical rethinking in neoconservative Britain.

The ideal underpinning community care is that people with health problems can be cared for in the community rather than in institutional settings. Policies aim to make appropriate caring services available both to those discharged from institutions, and to those who would otherwise have to move to institutions in order to receive the care they need. A successful programme of community care would be normalizing and integrative, rather than stigmatizing and segregative. It would create the conditions for sick people to participate fully in public life and to exercize their full range of citizenship rights. It would prevent people having to move home (which is always stressful and can be distressing) simply to ensure that they receive a particular package of medical services and social support. In theory, therefore, the development of community care could reduce pressures on the medical priority route into public sector housing, it could capitalize on the greater flexibility of health service provision envisaged in the National Health Service review, and in doing so, it could secure a range of basic social entitlements for people with health needs.

In principle then, the Griffiths report of 1988, and the white paper *Caring for People* (Secretaries of State for Health, Wales, Northern Ireland and Scotland 1989b) which followed it were widely welcomed. Here was the opportunity for community care to play a crucial meditating role between housing provision, medical needs, and access to health care services. The white paper did, moreover, offer a clear framework and a set of general principles which should help local authorities develop more coherent planning processes. In developing these plans local authorities will have to provide needs assessments for their local populations, they will need to specify arrangements for assessing the individuals who may be eligible for caring services, they will be required to draw up detailed budgeting arrangements, and they will be asked to indicate how the social service (which will take the lead role in developing community care) will be coordinated with the plans of health authorities, Family Health Service Authorities and the housing authorities.

Like the NHS white paper, *Caring for People* envisages a separation between service design and purchase from service provision, it demands a shift towards the management of services by contract and the development of a mixed economy of care; it places emphasis on accountability and forecasts the development of information systems for case management and costing (Murphy 1990). The new community care proposals thus bring the same reservations, as well as the same opportunities, as the new proposals for the NHS. Nevertheless, the new proposals seem in line with the development of policies for community care which, at a formal level, link housing provision with medical needs and the caring services.

In practice, however, the optimism that accompanies the new proposals is tempered on a number of grounds. Eyles (1988) puts the latest round of legislation in context by pointing out that the development of community care—however desirable and beneficial it may be—has always had a strong economic motive. It has always aimed to cut costs by shifting the burden of care to the informal sector. Even throughout the 1960s, the emphasis of community care was squarely on closing hospital beds rather than on providing facilities for care in the community. By the 1970s, the Government was planning to reduce rather than expand the proportion of the social security budget spent on personal social services. And despite a renewed commitment to community care in the 1980s—signalled by the publication of *Care in action* (Department of Health and Social Security 1981)—no new resources were made available and all community based facilities had to be funded out of local authorities' existing cash allowance.

In 1988, the House of Commons Social Services Committee announced that (for the first time in the postwar period) there would be a real decline in personal social services expenditure for the early 1990s. The same cost cutting principles appear in the 1990 white paper and in the legislation based on it, which will not now be implemented until April 1993. The evidence is therefore consistent with Eyles (1988) view that:

> Community care has become the dominant option, at least at the level of policy intention, because of its apparent cost-effectiveness, which is

in large measure ensured by not putting a financial value on the contributions of informal care-givers.... (p. 48).

Certainly, there are indications that home care is cheaper than institutional care, and that it may be preferable to many patients (Creese and Fielden 1977): but this line of argument tends to undervalue and undercost the role of carers. Carers may already save the state over £11 billion each year in service provision, but most observers agree that this level of commitment cannot be sustained, let alone increased, without better support services. As Walker (1987) points out, effective informal networks of care are unlikely to be created through welfare cuts.

In addition to the burden on carers, there is cause for concern about the extent to which service coordination will be achieved via the new proposals, and in particular, it is still apparent that the role of housing as an element of community care is underestimated and poorly thought through. Integrate (1990), for instance, call for housing agencies to have statutory rights and duties to participate on an equal basis in community care planning, jointly with social work/social service departments and health authorities/boards. They see housing as much more than bricks and mortar and argue that community care services should involve housing based initiatives such as care and repair schemes, alarms and adaptations (see also Harrison and Means 1990). Others are concerned about the potentially weak links between social services and housing, on the one hand—both functioning under the auspices of the local authorities—and the health services, on the other hand, administered through the health authorities, boards and trusts. Glennerster et al (1990) thus argue that health centres and budget holding general practitioners could also receive funding for community care initiatives.

All these ideas are interesting and stimulating, but it appears that any further innovations will be limited by costs. No new money is to be made available for the reforms to community care: changes will be funded simply by transferring (through a mechanism and in an amount which remains to be specified) part of the social security budget to the local authorities. As Glennerster et al (1990) point out:

> The central, if disguised, purpose behind the white paper is to check the rise in that part of the social security budget that has come to be devoted to the care of old people and others in private and voluntary homes (p 3).

This emphasis on cost cutting is what has produced most reservations with the new legislation. Many fear that service provision will be selective and that groups excluded will be forced to exchange the entitlements of their social contract for the vagaries of a commercial contract, where outcomes are determined less by need than by ability to pay. Langan (1990) fears the development of a two-tiered welfare system:

> In which the private and voluntary sectors look after anybody who can raise the required funds and the local authority deals with a residuum of the poorest, the most disturbed and the most difficult (p. 64).

She predicts an increasing reliance on the voluntary sector which will exacerbate inequalities in access to care—given that voluntary services are less available in poorer areas, and so are distributed in inverse proportion to need. And she concludes that the new legislation gives

> No real consideration to the question of how to empower the consumers of services, how to guarantee and extend the rights of all citizens to decent standards of care, how to ensure redress for the service user who is dissatisfied with the service provided. (p 68)

Her point is that not only might the new proposals continue to compromize the entitlements of those with health needs, but that they also deny the rights of carers. As Finch (1988) has argued:

> Women must have the right not to care, and dependent people must have the right not to rely on their relatives (p 30).

Putting it all together

As the twentieth century dawned, housing and health issues were inextricably linked at all levels of policy making. It was taken as axiomatic that housing impinged on illness and disease and that housing interventions were a route to better public health. In the intervening years, housing and health policies have gone their separate ways, and since the 1950s there have been few explicit links between the two areas at the level of legislation or in policy implementation. As the new millenium approaches, strategies for housing provision and health care servicing are being radically reappraised, and there is enormous potential for harnessing their points of intersection to ensure that sick people have a right to a decent home, and to ensure that people in any residential setting can exercise their right to health care. Sadly, there are few real signs that these points of contact are being developed.

The main role for housing policy in disease prevention and health promotion in recent years has been concerned with assigning medical priority to needy applicants in the queues for public sector housing. However, as we have seen, the scope for using rehousing as a general prescription for better health (or even for a better quality of life for a given health status) is diminishing. Rehousing is only a viable strategy where there is a relatively large pool of generally high quality dwellings available to housing managers. If the council sector continues to be a 'residual' sector, it is unlikely to be able to fill this role to any substantial extent.

This role for housing provision in meeting medical needs is, however, multifaceted: it involves moving people out of unhealthy homes into healthy ones; it involves moving people out of unsuitable homes into more suitable ones; it may be concerned with moving people to places where they have better access to health care and social support; and it sometimes includes provision for moving carers and those they care for so that the two can live closer together. Currently, the nature and effectiveness of using the medical priority system to fulfil these various roles is underresearched. There may well be value in enhancing the medical priority element of housing management, and in ensuring that the public sector housing stock is able to offer real choice to people with medical needs. However, there are also obvious ways in which a complementary suite of housing and health policies could address some of these issues outside (and alongside) the traditional medical priority system.

A public health perspective could, for instance, be invoked to monitor the health effects of housing interventions, and to target where housing improvements—in any sector of the housing system—could be most beneficial in public health terms. This could be as effective as rehousing in achieving the first aim listed above. The housing finance and benefits system could be returned to ensure that homes are adequately adapted for people with medical needs, to prevent people needing to move simply because they cannot fully use their existing dwellings. Reductions in inequalities in health service availability and delivery would make place of residence a less crucial determinant of access to health care: in the short term, this would benefit homeless people as well as those in more secure accommodation. A suite of housing policies geared more closely to the aims of community care would make rehousing unnecessary for many people who need intensive servicing. This could extend carers' rights as well as giving sick people an entitlement to independent living.

Our aim here is not to explore the alternatives in detail, but rather to point out that alternatives are available and that options do remain, even in a period of fiscal austerity. The relationships between housing, health and the caring services are not the product of chance: they are, rather, a product of political will. They are the endpoint of a series of decisions in a context where more than one outcome is usually possible. As Eyles (1988) notes when discussing the health services response to Britain's fiscal crisis:

> While this crisis, through the introduction of cash limits, helped to inaugurate a financially restricted restructuring of care, it was the social aims and philosophical rationale of the New Right that ensured that the restructuring would occur in the form and way it did (p 53).

There is nothing inevitable about the role of housing in health policy, or about the place of health concerns in housing policy. The link between housing and health—in policy and in practice—depends crucially on what role the public of Britain's 'postwelfare' state want housing policy to play in maintaining public health and sustaining social welfare.

References

Albertsen N 1988 Postmodernism, post-fordism and critical social theory. *Environment and Planning D: Society and Space* **6**: 339–65

Audit Commission 1986a *Managing the crisis in council housing.* HMSO, London

Audit Commission 1986b *Making a reality of community care.* HMSO, London

Beck E J, Adam S A Eds 1990 *The white paper and beyond.* Oxford University Press, Oxford

Bury B 1990 We will pick up the pieces, but...*British Medical Journal* **300**: 1083

Clapham D, Kemp P, Smith S J 1990 *Housing and social policy.* Macmillan, Basingstoke and London

Community Health Resource Unit (1990) Some good points from the white paper 'Working for patients'. *Community Health* **7**: 1–2

Creese A L and Fielden R 1977 Hospital or home care for the severely disabled: a cost comparison. *British Journal of Preventive and Social Medicine* **31**: 116–21

Crook A D H 1986 Privatisation of housing and the impact of the conservative Government's initiatives on low-cost home ownership and private renting between 1979 and 1984 in England and Wales: 1 The privatisation policies. *Environment and Planning A* **18**: 639–59

Deakin N 1987 *The politics of welfare* Methuen, London

Eyles J 1988 Mental health services, the restructuring of care, and the fiscal crisis of the state: the United Kingdom case study. *In* Smith C J, Giggs, J A Eds *Location and stigma.* Unwin Hyman, Boston, 36–57

Finch J 1988 Whose responsibility? Women and the future of family care. In Allen I, Wicks M, Finch J, Leat D Eds. *Informal care tomorrow* Policy Studies Institute, London

Ford J C 1990 General practice fundholders *British Medical Journal* **300**: 1027–28

Forrest R, Murie A 1988 *Selling the welfare state: the privatisation of public housing.* Routledge and Kegan Paul, London

Glennerster H, Falkingham J, Evandrou M 1990 How much do we care? A comment on the Government's community care proposals. *Welfare State Programme Discussion Paper* **46**: Centre for Economics and Related Disciplines, London School of Economics

Griffiths Report 1988 *Community care: agenda for action.* HMSO, London

Harrison L, Means R 1900 *Housing. The essential element in community care.* Anchor Housing Trust, Oxford

Harvey D 1989 *The condition of postmodernity.* Blackwell, Oxford

Integrate 1990 *Care for people. Policy statement.* Integrate, Glasgow

Jessop B 1988 Conservative regimes and the transition to post-fordism: the case of Britain and West Germany. *Papers in Politics and Government* **47**: Department of Government, University of Essex

Keane J 1988 *Democracy and civil society.* Verso, London

Kearns A 1990 *Voluntarism, management and accountability.* Housing Association Research Unit, University of Glasgow

Kearns A, Smith S J 1990 Housing studies of the New Times: on post-fordism and postmodernism. *Discussion Paper No.32*, Centre for Housing Research, Glasgow University

Langan M 1990 Community care in the 1990s: The community care white paper: 'Caring for people'. *Critical Social Policy* 10, 58–70

Lash S, Urry J 1987 *The end of organised capitalism* Polity Press, Cambridge

Malpass P, Murie A 1982 *Housing policy and practice.* Macmillan, London

Murphy E 1990 Meeting the needs of the most vulnerable. In Beck E J, Adam S A Eds *The white paper and beyond.* Oxford University Press, Oxford, 78–87

O'Donnell O 1989 *Mental health care policy in England: Objectives, failures and reforms.* Centre for Health Economics, University of York

Paton C 1990 The Prime Minister's review of the National Health Service and the 1989 white paper 'Working for patients'. In Manning N, Ungerson C Eds. *Social Policy Review 1989–90.* Longman, London

Plant R 1989 Can there be a right to health care? *Occasional paper*, Department of Politics, University of Southampton

Secretaries of State for Health, Wales, Northern Ireland and Scotland 1989a *Working for patients* CM555 HMSO, London

Secretaries of State for Health, Wales, Northern Ireland and Scotland 1989b *Caring for people* CM849 HMSO, London

Smith R 1987 *Unemployment and health.* Oxford University Press, Oxford

Smith S J 1989a Social geography: social policy and the restructuring of welfare. *Progress in Human Geography* **13**: 118–28

Smith S J 1989b Housing and health: review and research agenda. *Discussion Paper* **27**. Centre for Housing Research. Glasgow University.

SMith S J 1990 Health status and the housing system. *Social Science and Medicine* **31**: 753–62

Walker A 1987 Enlarging the caring capacity of the community: informal support networks and the welfare state. *International Journal of Health Services* **17**: 369–86

Weller M P I 1989 Mental illness-who cares? *Nature* **339**: 249–52

Index

AIDS and HIV
    housing needs, 114-16
    housing policy, 8-9
    housing provision, 112-13, 116-19
    specialist housing, 118
AIDS and Housing Project, 114
alcoholism, 155, 186, 187, 189, 191, 211, 214
antenatal care, 156,160, 161, 164, 176,
autism, 126

bed and breakfast
    accommodation, 12, 168, 180-83
    access to health care, 176-78
    conditions, 168, 170-72
    health problems, 75, 111, 164, 174-78
Beveridge report, 155
Black report, 155

Canada, 204
cardiovascular/neurological
    disorders, 76, 190, 191
carers, 7, 25, 120, 121, 139, 227, 228, 229
Caring for People white
    paper, 134-36, 140, 149, 225-6
child abuse, 155
children, 2, 35, 67, 157, 164, 176-77
circulatory disorders, 77, 190
community care, 10, 120-21, 134, 225-27
    housing and, 128-34, 134-40, 225-26
    'special' policies, 137, 139, 149
community health services, 24-5, 29-30

Cumberlege report, 31-2

damp, 1-2, 65, 74, 75, 78, 111, 157
diet, 169, 171-73, 177-78
disability, 76, 77, 134
    adaptation of dwellings, 63, 66, 101, 136
    homelessness, 94,
    housing needs, 7-8, 35, 77-8, 93
    housing policy, 67, 93-103, 109-13
    independent living, 104-8
    rehousing, 84-5
    rights, 91
    tenure, 93-5

elderly, 38, 67, 77 94, 102, 123-24, 134, 137
ethnic minorities, 23, 31, 32, 35, 38
    discrimination, 93
    homelessness, 157
    housing policy, 97
Family Health Service
Authorities (FHSAs), 24, 27
general practitioner services
    access, 25-9, 37, 46, 156, 176-77, 196-98
    quality, 30-2
    budgets, 199, 223-24
Great Chapel Street Medical
    Centre, 186-90
Griffiths report, 135, 147-48, 225

'Health Field Concept of
    Health', 75
high rise flats, 174
homelessness, 10-13, 80, 184
    access to health care, 156-57, 195-99, 223
    health effects, 67-9, 76,